Sacred Rites for Rejuvenation

Sacred Rites
for Rejuvenation

Samael Aun Weor

Sacred Rights for Rejuvenation
A Glorian Book

© 2018 Glorian Publishing

Print ISBN: 978-1-934206-79-9
Ebook ISBN: 978-1-934206-84-3

Glorian Publishing is a non-profit organization.
All proceeds go to further the distribution
of these books. For more information, visit
gnosticteachings.org.

Contents

Editor's Introduction

The following text is transcribed from oral instructions given by Samael Aun Weor to a student. The transcribed text was initially published by that student decades ago in Spanish in the form of a narrative, and included many personal anecdotes and writings unrelated to the teachings. In later years, other Gnostic students decided to publish an edition that removed the extraneous material, resulting in a series of completely unrelated chapters. In 2008, Glorian Publishing translated and published the first English edition of that book. However, new readers were very confused by the jumbled collection of chapters, causing many to believe that Samael Aun Weor wrote the book in that form, which reflected badly on the teachings. In this edition, we have removed the extraneous chapters and focused entirely on the practical rites. For those who are interested in reading the other chapters, they are available as online articles at gnosticteachings.org.

Furthermore, this book should not be read as an introduction to the teachings, nor even as a thorough explanation of the exercises themselves. These exercises come from an ancient, protected tradition whose full depth can be accessed only by those who put these exercises into practice and awaken their consciousness.

To learn about Gnosis, the teachings of Samael Aun Weor, and awakening consciousness, visit gnosticteachings.org.

Yantra Yoga

The Sanskrit word yantra implies "restraint" or "firm support," and can literally be translated as "machine, instrument." The word yantra has different implications depending upon which tradition is using it.

In Hinduism, this term is usually used in Hindu Tantra (esoteric teachings) in reference to mystical diagrams or forms utilized in meditation.

In Buddhism, yantra refers to a series of bodily movements taught in Buddhist Tantra to specially prepared students. The Indian Tantric Master Padmasambhava and his student, a Tibetan scholar and monk named Vairochana, are credited with establishing Buddhism in Tibet (especially Dzogchen) in the eighth century A.D., as well as setting the foundations for Tibetan medicine and a highly sophisticated series

of physical and energetic exercises called
"Yantra Yoga" (Tibetan: 'khrul 'khor)
whose purpose was to establish a strong
foundation for spiritual development.
Today, these exercises are practiced in some
of the schools of Tibetan Buddhism, but
kept only amongst the initiated. As Samael
Aun Weor said in the following book,
some of these exercises have been described
publicly, but in an incomplete form.

The true Yantric exercises have some
relationship with Hatha Yoga (now very
popular in the West), Chi Gung, and various
martial arts, all of which originated with the
intention of keeping the physical body fit
enough to withstand the intense demands
of spiritual development. Clearly, Hatha
Yoga and the martial arts have largely
forgotten their spiritually-focused roots,
the evidence of which is their complete
inability to awaken the consciousness of
their practitioners. The exercises described
in this book, however, are very different,
and when practiced faithfully, can awaken
the consciousness and provide many other
essential benefits.

Among the Tibetan Buddhist schools,
there are several variations and lineages of
Yantra Yoga. The exercises taught in this

book are drawn from but not identical to those traditions. As stated herein:

> "These rites are not the exclusive patrimony of anyone. There are some monasteries in the Himalayas and in other places where these rites are practiced, mainly in a monastery that is called 'The Fountain of Youth'...
>
> "I obtained some data from the mentioned monastery, which I know very well, and other data from other schools in India that I also know very well."

The Authenticity of the Author

Between 1950 and 1977, a mere twenty-seven years, Samael Aun Weor (which is a Hebrew name) wrote over sixty books (seventy if you include collections of lectures), gave thousands of lectures, and formed the worldwide Gnostic Movement, whose members number in the millions. Though these accomplishments are certainly impressive by any standard, they are merely the pale, terrestrial reflection of the work he accomplished internally, spiritually. And yet, in spite of his wisdom and generosity towards mankind, he said:

"Do not follow me. I am just a signpost. Reach your own Self-realization."

His lifelong mission was to deliver to humanity the complete path toward the realization of the inner Being, or in other words, the total and exact science required by anyone of any religion, race, culture or creed who wishes to fully and completely develop the human potential.

"When the mind is quiet, when the mind is silent—that is, when the mind is empty of thoughts, desires, opinions, etc.—then, the truth comes into us.

"To arrive at the experience of reality is only possible when all thoughts have ceased.

"The eruption of the Void allows us to experience the bright light of pure reality.

"That ever-present knowledge, which in reality is empty, without characteristics or color, devoid of condition, is the true reality, the universal compassion.

"Your intelligence, whose true nature is the Void—which must not be seen as a void of nothingness, but as that very intelligence without shackles: brilliant, universal, and happy—is Cognizance, the Buddha, universally wise.

"Your own empty cognizance and that brilliant and joyful intelligence are inseparable; their union forms the Dharmakaya, the state of perfect illumination.

"Your own brilliant cognizance, empty and inseparable from the great body of splendor, has neither birth nor death: it is the immutable light, the Amitaba Buddha.

"This knowledge is enough. To recognize the emptiness of your own intelligence as the Buddhic state and to consider it as your own cognizance is to continue within the divine spirit of Buddha." —Samael Aun Weor, *Fundamentals of Gnostic Education* (1970)

The path he taught to achieve this knowledge is that of the Bodhisattva, that mysterious and ancient wisdom long hidden in the bosom of every great religion.

> *"For as long as space endures and for as long as the world lasts, may I live dispelling the miseries of the world."* —Shantideva, *The Guide to the Bodhisattva's Way of Life*

The Bodhisattva path, also known as the straight path, is taken by very few.

While many aspire to the Light, the vast majority take the easier spiral path, which is accomplished over a much longer period. The walker of the straight path is rare because that road is bitter, painful, and filled with terrors, yet is the only one capable of reaching the Ultimate. Embodied in the life story of many masters, including Jesus of Nazareth, the path of the Bodhisattva is a path of self-sacrifice on behalf of others.

> "The straight path, the upright course of action, the eightfold path, conducts us from the darkness to the light. Thus, this is what Christ meant when he said to us: "I am the way, the truth, and the life: no man cometh unto the Father, but by me." (John 14:6)

> "Those who renounce the happiness of Nirvana because of their love for mankind, those who have the body or vehicle of solar transformation, the Nirmanakaya, are the authentic Bodhisattvas, who indeed walk along the straight path; they know the word of the Lord.

> "Regarding myself, concerning me, I am a walker of the straight path; thus, I teach the doctrine related with the

straight path for those who want to go on the straight path." —Samael Aun Weor

Clearly, the path taught by Samael Aun Weor is a radical departure from the teachings of the spiral path, and is even more sharply opposed to the far more common teachings of "the Baalim," the lunar path, which Jesus called wide and broad, or easy to follow.

> *"Therefore all things whatsoever ye would that men should do to you, do ye even so to them: for this is the law and the prophets.*
>
> *"Enter ye in at the strait gate: for wide [is] the gate, and broad [is] the way, that leadeth to destruction, and many there be whch go in thereat:*
>
> *"Because strait [is] the gate, and narrow [is] the way, which leadeth unto life, and few there be that find it."* —Matthew 7

Millions of religious followers think they have found the true way, but the great Master Jesus said that only a few find the way to "life."

Thus, the student, when encountering the teachings of the straight path for the first time, is often shocked, outraged, or offended, because these teachings contradict much of what we believe or hold dear. Upon closer study, it will be discovered that Gnosis is indeed the doctrine of synthesis, the expression of the universal wisdom in the heart of every religion. What is in conflict with Gnosis are the ideas and interpretations of mankind. Truth is one; it is our mind that degenerates that truth into opinions, dogmas, politics, and wars.

As a vibrant embodiment of the Bodhisattva ideal, which renounces all self-interest and seeks instead to benefit others, Samael Aun Weor rejected any notion of personality worship or the attachments of followers. Throughout his life, many thousands of students projected onto him their ideals and their needs, and this continues to this day. While many worship him and make Gnosis into just another system of belief, his own message is very clear: the only Master we should follow is our own inner Divinity. To reach that inner Divinity, we must remove from our mind mere belief: we must instead study the path as taught by all the great teachers of humanity, and put those teachings into daily practice.

Perhaps most remarkably, what he wrote and taught was not mere theory:

unlike most authors (especially those who write about religion and spirituality), he taught from personal experience.

> "There are authors who write marvels, but when one looks at them, one realizes that they have not lived what they have written; they did not experience it in themselves, and that is why they are mistaken. I understand that one must write what one has directly experienced by oneself. For my part, I have proceeded in this way."
> —Samael Aun Weor, *Tarot and Kabbalah* (1978)

The techniques in this book reflect the profound, core teachings hidden in many religions. Samael Aun Weor explains that these techniques are derived from Tibetan, India, Middle Eastern, and Latin American sources. Nevertheless, their primary source is Tibetan Tantra. Remarkably, these techniques were taught in Latin America in the mid-twentieth century, at a time when the various lineages of Tibetan Buddhism were scrambling to survive being purged from the planet. During those decades, only a handful of genuine Tibetan scriptures were available outside of closed circles, and those few scriptures were poorly translated, incomplete, and not very revealing, especially regarding actual techniques. Furthermore, they were

not available in Latin America, where
Samael Aun Weor resided. Nevertheless,
during those decades Samael Aun Weor
wrote detailed explanations of the very
core philosophies and techniques of the
highest forms of Tibetan Buddhism, yet
he did so in the language of his readers so
they would understand (that is, he did not
pepper his writings with terms that would
be unknown or obscure to them). However,
those who know the Tibetan teachings can
now read those writings and see very clearly
that Samael Aun Weor not only knew the
Dharma in depth, but knew intimate details
of Tibetan Buddhism that were never
published anywhere, even amongst many
levels of study in the Tibetan schools.

It has often been asked how he acquired
his knowledge. Samael Aun Weor stated
that he was a reincarnated Tibetan lama,
but he never gave details about his Tibetan
background, because he was not interested
in impressing anyone or convincing
anyone to follow him. Instead, he only
wanted humanity to practice the Dharma.
Therefore, to understand who he is and how
he knew what he wrote, he always advised
his students to awaken consciousness for
themselves.

Terminology

These exercises have been known by various names, notably called by Gnostic students "the Tibetan rites" or "the lamasery exercises." It is important to note that the term "lamasery" did not originate in Asia, but was invented by Westerners. Samael Aun Weor used the term as was conventional at the time he was teaching. However, in the spirit of continual improvement that he followed, and with respect to the tradition from which these exercises are derived, we prefer not to perpetuate the use of the term. Therefore, in this book we have exchanged the misnomer "lamasery" for the more accurate and appropriate term "monastery."

Prologue

During the moments in which I write this prologue, before my sight within this park of the capital city of Mexico, I observe some people seated on benches contemplating the beauties of nature: beautiful trees, gorgeous fields, and some children playing in the warm rays of the sun.

Many scenes emerge from within my memory... dramas, extraordinary events from ancient times, like: initiatic colleges, solitary hermitages, where, amidst singing rivulets running precipitately along their bed of rocks, the anchorites meditated in silence; marvelous Sibyls from the druids of Europe, and from primeval times, the hermits of the ancient Egypt of the Pharaohs, etc.

There is no doubt, brothers and sisters, that in those times of yore, within the mysteries of Eleusis, Troy, Rome, Carthage, Egypt, etc., the psychological and the physical marched in a harmonious, perfect, parallel way.

For instance, in these moments I remember the Pythagorean mysteries to which, in ancient times, those who lacked mathematical knowledge were not admitted.

Remember the whirling dervishes, the magnificent runes, the beautiful dances of India, the perfect rhythmical movements of the Egyptian initiates: in them all you will see, brothers and sisters, the extraordinary parallel that has always has been there between the spiritual, the psychological, and the physical.

Indubitably, we have a body of bones and flesh; that body possesses a marvelous eurhythmy, and within the brain there are many latent powers that must be awakened. Thus, it is indispensable to learn how to handle our body, to know how to take, to extract, the sweetest melodies from it. It is important to make it vibrate as a symphony of the miraculous harp of the universe.

It is absurd, my beloved brothers and sisters, to allow Heropass [time] to damage this precious physical vehicle, which has been granted unto us for the realization of our Inner Self.

Verily, I tell you, brothers and sisters, that we, the Gnostics, have precise methods in order to rejuvenate the organism and cure all sicknesses. It is unquestionable that we can learn how to heal ourselves. Each one of us can be converted into our own physician by learning how to heal ourselves without the necessity of "medicine"—lo and behold, the most beloved ideal.

It is urgent to preserve the physical body in perfect health for many years so that we can use this precious physical vehicle for the realization of our Inner Self.

Here we deliver the necessary exercises for the preservation of health and for the prolongation of life. Here you have, brothers and sisters, the precious methods by means of which you (if you are old) can re-conquer youth, and if you are young, can prolong that youth indefinitely.

Therefore, understand by reading with attention, and then practice. It would be worthless for you to just theorize, thus it is necessary to go to the point, straight to the facts, because this is simultaneously an eminently practical and didactical book.

These teachings are delivered in a dialectical way. However, I repeat, do not become content only with bookish information: transform the doctrine into facts, because the teachings that we deliver in this book are also for the awakening of the consciousness.

Yes, the hour, the moment, has arrived for the awakening of the consciousness; why should we continue with our consciousness asleep, when the one hundred percent efficient and absolutely practical procedures for awakening are delivered in this book?

Thus, if each of the devotees practices meditation in the manner that we have taught, they will then, any day, reach Samadhi.[1]

Now, with the precise didactical and practical exercises given, any sincere aspirant can provoke the great permutation—that is, authentic, radical transformation.

First of all, what is indeed most essential is to have a continuity of purpose: it is not enough to practice today, and forget about it tomorrow. Thus, it is necessary to practice and to practice intensely for our entire life until reaching the goal: the ultimate triumph.

---

1   "... a transcendental state of wonderment, which is associated with perfect mental clarity." See glossary for full definition.

May peace be with all of humanity.
Samael Aun Weor

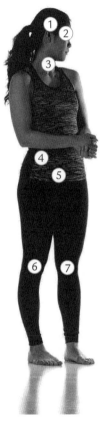

THE SEVEN CHAKRAS RELATED TO ORGANIC VITALITY

The Sacred Rites

It is necessary to know that in our human body, in our cellular organism, we have some chakras[2] that we can qualify as specific, special for our organic vitality. They are like vortices through which Prana,[3] life, enters into our organism. They are, namely:

- First, the occipital [pineal gland]
- Second, the frontal [pituitary gland]
- Third, the laryngeal located at the throat [thyroid gland]
- Fourth, the hepatic [liver]
- Fifth, the prostatic / uterine
- Sixth and seventh are the two related chakras located at the knees

So, these are the seven basic chakras [related to organic vitality; there are additional chakras in the organism]; again, these are important for the vitality of our physical organism since through these chakras, the life, Prana, enters our vital

2 Subtle centers of energetic transformation. See glossary for full definition.
3 Life-principle; the breath of life; energy. See glossary for full definition.

body,[4] which is the seat of all organic activity.

For example, the laryngeal chakra [in the throat] maintains a close relation with the prostatic / uterine chakra; this is why what we say, our words, must be carefully weighed. Likewise, we need to carefully avoid making very low or shrieking sounds when we speak; i.e., if we carefully observe decrepit old people, we can easily verify that when they speak they emit sounds that we could perfectly call shrieking; these sounds corrupt their sexual potency, or accurately indicate impotency. The same occurs with sounds that are too deep or cavernous; these also corrupt the sexual potency. Therefore, the male's voice must remain within its normal range; likewise, the woman's voice must not be too low or shrieking, because this corrupts her sexual potency due to the intimate relationship between the larynx and the sexual center. The former statement could be challenged since the woman does not have a prostate. True, she does not have a prostate, yet she has a chakra

---

4   The superior aspect of the physical body, composed of the energy or vital force that provides life to the physical body. See glossary for full definition.

related to her uterus, and this plays a very important role in her body, as important as the prostatic chakra in the man. In the woman, we could call this chakra the uterine chakra, and we already know the importance of the uterus in the woman.

After this short preamble, and as a matter of information, for the benefit of our Gnostic brothers and sisters we are going to narrate something of great significance.

It so happened that sometime ago in India there lived an English colonel who was about seventy years old. He was retired from active military service and had a young friend. The colonel heard about a monastery of lamas[5] in Tibet where old people become young, in other words, where many who arrived old left young. The method to accomplish this is something that I will transcribe later in a precise manner for all of you. At this moment I only want to explain how these six rites make it possible to bring back youth, which was the concern of the English colonel.

---

5   A title used in Tibetan Buddhism for a teacher of religion.

First of all, we must always seek to be in good health, because a healthy body is good for everything, withstands everything, and responds at all moments so that we can demand from it our material and spiritual work. So, the first thing, as I already stated, is to cure the body and to maintain its resistance throughout our entire lifetime. Therefore, we must maintain it in good condition, because what can one do with a sick body? It is obvious that an esotericist, an initiate, must never be sick; illnesses and tormenting problems are for people who are not on the real path, is it not so? Indeed, those who are on the path should neither be decrepit nor sick; this is clear.

Therefore, this is why there is a series of very important esoteric exercises; i.e. much has been stated in esotericism, in Kundalini Yoga,[6] about the Viparitakarani Mudra, likewise about the dancing dervishes or whirling dervishes. In Pakistan, in India, etc., the dervishes know how to execute certain marvelous dances in order

6   The method to awaken the intelligence of the Divine Mother within oneself, called Kundalini, candali, pentecost, etc. and represented by the ubiquitous serpent of mythology that accompanies Moses, Hermes, Athena, etc.

to awaken certain faculties, powers, or chakras. Thus, it is urgent to know all of this if we want to have a youthful body and to develop the chakras. Therefore, let us study this series of exercises.

Young people do not appreciate the value of youth because they are young, yet old people do appreciate the treasure of youth. Thus, with the practices of the six rites that we will demonstrate, an old person can rejuvenate; in other words, if the person is old, he or she can recapture their youth. It is clear that if the person is young, he or she can remain young by means of these rites.

Any person can cure his pains with these exercises; among them, we will show here:

· Mayurasana

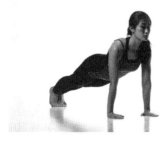

· the kneeling position

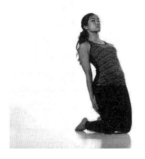

· the table posture that is shown
  in some sacred ruins, etc.

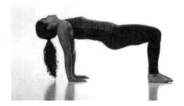

These are a synthesis of esoteric
exercises, documented in India, Persia,
Pakistan, Turkey, Yucatan, Mexico, etc.

I have read some of the publications
out there; regrettably, they do not teach
the fully equilibrated formula as it should
necessarily be. Therefore, what I am going
to teach to all of you is very important

and it must be very well taught in South America and to all the brothers and sisters of the Gnostic Movement, so that old people can become youthful again; Gnostics who are seventy years old can, for example, become as if they were thirty-five or forty years old.

Some will question why I do not look younger. I will answer them that it is simply because I was not interested in preserving this physical body, but now, as I was informed that I could conserve this body for an indefinite time in order to initiate the Age of Aquarius,[7] it is obvious that for this reason I have to practice these exercises.

Sometime ago I read a publication that had these rites in it; this was sent to me from Costa Rica. Notwithstanding, these rites are not the exclusive patrimony of anyone.

There are some monasteries in the Himalayas and in other places where these rites are practiced, mainly in a monastery that is called "The Fountain of Youth";

7 An era of time under the influence of the zodiacal sign of Aquarius that will last for approximately 2,140 years. The new Aquarian era began with the celestial conjunction of February 4-5, 1962.

however, even though many exercises are practiced there, I did not find the complete documentation of these exercises in the above-mentioned publication. I obtained some data from the mentioned monastery, which I know very well, and other data from other schools in India that I also know very well.

When one takes the trouble of traveling a little through Turkey, Persia, Pakistan, etc., then one can learn something about the dancing or whirling dervishes, etc.

We need to reflect a little about what being on one's knees symbolizes, since when one is a child, one unconsciously practices certain exercises.

Now, I am going to continue the very intriguing narration that I read in that publication, which is the very interesting story of that English colonel that I am going to write in detail so that all of you can have an exact and complete idea about the benefits that are acquired with the exercises that I am teaching here.

In the above-mentioned magazine, they wrote of the case of that seventy-year-old English colonel, who learned in India of the existence of a monastery in Tibet where people could rejuvenate. He invited a friend to come along with him. Yet, since his friend was young, obviously he did not listen; the young man would have thought why should he go in search for a place to rejuvenate since he was already young.

On the day of the wretched old-man's departure, his young friend—as is to be expected—laughed a great deal when seeing the wretched seventy-year-old man with his cane, bald head, a few white hairs, very old, traveling towards the Himalayas in search of youth. In the mind of his young friend the following thoughts arose: "How funny is this old man: he already lived his life and wants to live it again." Thus, he saw the old man leaving and the only thing it caused in him was laughter.

Interestingly, after about four months, the colonel's young friend received a letter from the old man in which he was informed that the colonel was already on the track of the monastery called "The Fountain of Youth." This, of course, caused only laughter to the young man; thus this subject-matter lingered.

Then, indeed, four years later, something happened that was no longer a laughing matter. Someone presented himself at the house of the young man and knocked on the door. The young man opened the door and said, "At your service; what can I do for you?"

The visitor, who appeared to be a man about thirty-five to forty-years old, answered, "I am colonel so-and-so."

"Ah...," said the young man, "Are you the son of the colonel who left for the Himalayas?"

The visitor answered, "No! I am the colonel himself."

The young man answered, "That is not possible. I know the colonel; he is my friend. He is an old man and you are not old."

The visitor answered, "I repeat: I am the colonel who wrote you a letter four months after my departure. In it I informed you that I had found the way to the monastery."

Thereafter, the visitor showed his documentation to his young friend; indeed, his young friend was astounded.

What is intriguing about this is that during his time in the Himalayas in that monastery called "The Fountain of Youth," the colonel saw many youths with whom he established friendships. There was not a single old person in that monastery; everybody was young. He was the only old person; all the others were people between thirty-five and forty years of age. However, after a while, when he had become very good friends with many of them, he discovered that all of them were more than one hundred years old. In other words, all of them surpassed his age, but none of them appeared as an old person. Obviously, the colonel was astounded, and thus he dedicated himself to the discipline of that monastery and succeeded in re-conquering his youth.

Well, I read the entire story in that publication they sent me. Nevertheless, I personally know that monastery: I have been there; it is a very large building with immense courtyards. The males work in one courtyard and the female initiates in another. The female initiates in that monastery are not only Tibetan women, but English, French, German, and women from other European countries.

Since ancient times, I have known all the exercises that are taught in that monastery. I.e.:

· I have long known the whirling
  movements of the Mohammedans;
  these dances constitute part of the
  esoteric aspect of Mohammedanism
  and are practiced—as I already
  stated—by the whirling dervishes.

· As far as the kneeling position
  is concerned, that belongs to
  the special technical movements
  of esoteric mysticism.

· As for the table posture,
  this is found in Yucatan.

· As for the position which some
  call the lizard posture —which is
  an exercise meant to reduce the
  abdomen—it is documented in
  Hindustan, in Kundalini Yoga,
  and is simply called Mayurasana.

· The laying position with
  perpendicular legs (upward feet)
  has abundant documentation.
  This has always been known as
  the Viparitakarani Mudra; we
  find it in many sacred texts.

· Likewise, the famous Vajroli
  Mudra, which is useful for sexual
  transmutation for bachelors and

bachelorettes; Vajroli Mudra also helps a great deal those who work with the Sahaja Maithuna.

Many publications have been printed concerning this series of exercises, yet they are not the exclusive property of any person, and as I stated, few are those who know the esoteric part of them. I know the esoteric part of them, not merely because of what might be said in the mentioned publication from Costa Rica, or the many others publications that we have read and which have published these exercises, but because I have known them since a very long time ago.

Indeed, I have known these rites practically since Lemuria.[8] For example, I practiced the Viparitakarani Mudra intensely when I was reincarnated on the continent Mu or Lemuria; thus I know practically how very important this is.

---

8   "It is clear that the Miocene Epoch had its proper scenario on the ancient Lemurian land, the continent that was formerly located in the Pacific Ocean. Remnants of Lemuria are still located in Oceania, in the great Australia, and on Easter Island (where some carved monoliths were found), etc." —Samael Aun Weor, *Gnostic Anthropology*

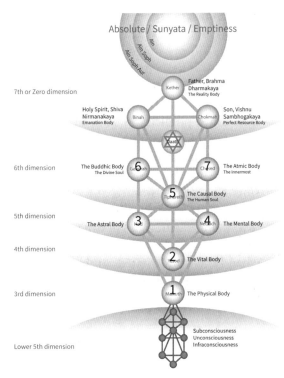

Absolute / Sunyata / Emptiness

Ain
Ain Soph
Ain Soph Aur

7th or Zero dimension

Father, Brahma
Dharmakaya
The Reality Body

Kether

Holy Spirit, Shiva
Nirmanakaya
Emanation Body

Binah

Son, Vishnu
Sambhogakaya
Perfect Resource Body

Chokmah

Daath

6th dimension

The Buddhic Body
The Divine Soul

6 Geburah

7 Chesed

The Atmic Body
The Innermost

5 Tiphereth

The Causal Body
The Human Soul

5th dimension

The Astral Body

3 Hod

4 Netzach

The Mental Body

4th dimension

2 Yesod

The Vital Body

3rd dimension

1 Malkuth

The Physical Body

Lower 5th dimension

Subconsciousness
Unconsciousness
Infraconsciousness

"THE HOLY SPIRIT" CORRESPONDS TO THE
SEPHIRAH BINAH ON THE TREE OF LIFE.

Healing Through the Intervention of the Holy Spirit

Let us now enter into the practical aspect of this matter; let us teach to the brothers and sisters of international Gnosticism everything that I deliver from the Patriarchal Headquarters of the Gnostic Movement in the capital city of Mexico.

It would please me very much if all of you learn these six rites that I am going to teach.

Indeed, I am going to teach you six rites. Understand that these are not merely physical calisthenics, no! These are RITES[9] practiced by the lamas who work in that monastery called "The Fountain of Youth." They use a prayer rug, which is a small rug on which they perform these rite-exercises; on it they lie down, they kneel, they sit, etc.

Meditation and prayer correspond with each posture or sadhana; in other

---

9   from Latin *ritus* "religious observance or ceremony, custom, usage."

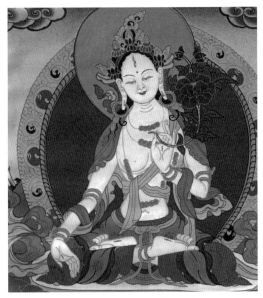

THE DIVINE MOTHER AS DEPICTED BY TIBETAN BUDDHISM

words, when they change a rite-posture, they intensify their meditation and prayer on any of the mystical aspects, in accordance to what they are beseeching for.

The Divine Mother Kundalini[10] is the central focal point of each sadhana.[11]

10 The feminine, receptive force through which creation occurs, symbolized in many religions by figures such as Isis, Mary, Maya, Tara, Isobertha, Rhea, Cybele, Gaea, etc. See the glossary.

11 "Instrument, means." A spiritual technique or method.

Thus, when we are performing these exercises, we must be in perfect concentration and prayer; we are beseeching, begging to the Divine Mother for our most urgent necessity. Through her, we can ask of the Logos.[12] She intercedes for us before the Logos. She pleads with us; she begs for us. She has great power, thus we beg to her, the Divine Mother, to intercede for us before the Third Logos,[13] so that she may beseech to the Logos for healing, for the awakening of our consciousness, the awakening of any chakra, etc.

Each position is different and each implies an intensification of our prayer, our petition, our pleading, our begging.

In these exercises of meditation, concentration, and pleading, we may very well ask our Divine Mother to invoke, by her will, her divine husband, the Third Logos, the very sacred Holy Spirit.[14] We already know very well that the husband of the Divine Mother is the Holy Spirit.

It is necessary to beg and to intensely beseech our Divine Mother so that she

---

12 "... the fundamental intelligent principle of nature." See the glossary.

13 The creative aspect of the universal trinity.

14 The Christian name for the third aspect of the Holy Trinity, or "God." See the glossary.

may, in turn, beg and beseech her divine
husband to heal us, and to relieve us
from any illness or pain that is afflicting
us. This way, she will concentrate in the
Logos, her husband, the arch-hierophant
or arch-magus (as he is named) so that he
may come and heal this or that sick organ
that is hindering the rendering of our
work.

In these moments, we must identify
ourselves as being one with the Logos,[15]
with the Holy Spirit and, in a tremendous, imperative way, we command the
sick organ saying:

Be healed! Be healed! Be healed! Work! Work! Work![16]

We must talk to the organ with true
faith, with energy, with courage, since it
has to unavoidably be healed.

We must definitely be concentrated
on each cell of the sick organ, on each
atom, on each molecule, on each electron
of the sick organ, and commanding it
to work, to be healed, to be cured, while

---

15   In tantric deity yoga, the practitioner imagines
     herself to be the deity she is invoking, and get
     the human personality out of the way.

16   All prayers and mantras like this can be recited
     mentally, that is, silently.

being profoundly concentrated on the Logos, completely identified as being one with the Holy Spirit, who in those moments is performing the cure, the healing of the sick organ. Thus, in this way, the organ will have to be healed, it will have to be cured; this is obvious.

Therefore, it is commendable for each person to learn how to cure himself. Through the strength of the Holy Spirit, we are able to cure ourselves; we are able to cure any illness.

This problem of going around sick is very depressing, very painful, and as I have already stated, those who walk on the path should not have the basis for being sick. So, these exercises develop the chakras and, on the other hand, they heal our organism.

There are very important chakras, i.e.:

· The one on the occipital [in the brain] is a door through which many forces enter into our organism.

· The frontal [between the eyebrows] is another door through which vital forces enter into the organism, when their chakras are developed.

· The larynx, as I have already stated, has an intimate relationship with the prostatic /uterine chakra, which is related with both sexes, the male and the female; thus, the prostatic/uterine as well as the larynx are very important for the health of our organism.

· Another is the chakra of the liver: as you know, the liver is a true laboratory. We must develop the hepatic chakra in order for the liver to function correctly, because when the liver is functioning well, subsequently the organism also functions well.

· There are also chakras of the knees. There are two, one on each knee, and these are vital for the human body. These vortices of strength must intensively spin in order for life—Prana, health—to enter into the human body.

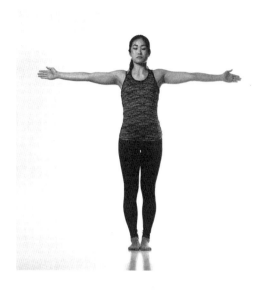

First Rite

Standing on their feet, the students extend their arms from side to side, forming the shape of a cross. Thereafter, they begin to turn around, to spin their body from left to right clockwise.

It is clear that the chakras will also spin with some intensity while performing this rite-exercise, and after some time of practice.

Let us imagine that we are standing in the center of a large clock; thus, we spin clockwise, in the same direction of the needles of the clock, until completing twelve turns. It is clear that some will begin with few turns, yet the day will arrive when they will completely perform all twelve turns.

We must whirl around with the eyes open, yet when we finish our turns, we must close our eyes in order to not fall, since we will be a little woozy according to the number of turns we are able to perform. Thus, one day we will be able to perform the complete exercise of twelve turns. Students will keep their eyes closed until the dizziness has disappeared.

Meanwhile, they will keep their prayer, their pleading, and imploration to their Divine Mother so that she may plead and beg her divine husband to grant us the healing of any particular sick organ. The student must be totally identified as being one with the Logos while intensely asking the Divine Mother for her intervention on behalf of the student before the Logos.

We have to spin clockwise from left to right, because amongst the mediums (channelers) of spiritualism, their chakras turn counterclockwise, from right to left, meaning in a negative way, and that way is useless. We, Gnostics, are not mediums or anything of the sort. Thus, we must develop our chakras in a positive manner.

Therefore, the system that I am teaching to all of you is marvelous, because it allows the development of the chakras and the healing of illnesses. All of the following rite-exercises complement each other.

We must start performing the exercise in a practical manner while concentrated on our Divine Mother Kundalini. Our feet must be together in military style, firm, arms extended from side to side.

Thereafter we begin to spin from left to right, while intensely asking for what we most need, above all, for the healing of the organ that may be sick, is it not? Thus, subsequently we may ask for our chakras to spin. It is clear that if we rotate clockwise, from left to right, in the same way as the needles of a clock that is seen, not on you, but in front of your sight, the chakras will rotate positively. Therefore, turn around and around at the rhythm that you consider convenient. Twelve turns is what is mandatory; however, if after you complete twelve, you want to continue up to thousand, well, that is up to you.

During the turns that we are performing, we must be concentrated on our Divine Mother Kundalini, asking her to call the Holy Spirit, thus imploring him to heal us, begging the Logos to cure us. Moreover, we must open the sick organ by pronouncing unto it:

> **Open Sesame!**[17]
> **Open Sesame!**
> **Open Sesame!**

This mantra[18] appears in the book *One Thousand and One Nights.* People think that book simply contains very beautiful tales. They do not pay attention to that mantra. Nevertheless, "Open Sesame" is an authentic mantra.

So, command the organ to open so that the healing vital energy will enter

---

17   The vowels are pronounced in their ancient forms: o as in "show," e as in "tell," and a as in "ball." The m and s are also considered mantric vowels and can be extended as mmmm and sssss.

18   Sanskrit, literally "mind protection." A sacred word or sound.

into you through it. Thus, this is how the
force of the Holy Spirit enters the sick
organ. It is clear that the organ becomes
healed with the force of the Third Logos.
Notwithstanding, we must execute all
of this with much faith, more faith, and
more faith.

Now, after your spinning exercise has
finished, open your eyes. Lie down on the
floor on your back—in other words, facing upwards—legs stretched out with your
heels together, your arms also stretched
but horizontally, extended from side to
side so that you make the form of the
cross with your body, looking upwards
towards the ceiling of the house.

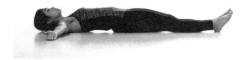

Here, you intensify your concentration. Intensify your meditation on the
Divine Mother Kundalini, begging her,
imploring her, to cure the sick organ
that you want to heal. Likewise, at that
moment, those who are not asking for

healing can ask for any other necessity, such as the elimination of any "I," any psychological defect or the development of any psychic power, etc. We have the right to ask, since this is the purpose of these exercises.

Thus, while lying down on your back on the floor, we supplicate and intensify our prayer, our petition, completely identifying ourselves as being one with the Third Logos. Therefore, the second position is to lie on the floor in the shape of a cross. We now know how to supplicate and ask in this position.

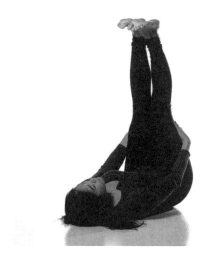

Second Rite

You have made your petitions while lying down in the shape of the cross; now raise your legs perpendicularly until they are in a vertical position. Here, it is no longer necessary to keep your arms extended and forming the horizontal line of the cross. So, move them so that with your hands you help to sustain your legs by holding them at the back of your knees, making sure that your legs are as vertical as possible without raising your buttocks from the floor, or more clearly stated, your waist must be very well placed on the floor, resting on the floor.

This is what in the East is called the Viparitakarani Mudra.[19] In this position, all the blood flows towards the head. It is precipitated towards the cranium so that determined areas of the brain can be set to work, likewise in order to fortify the senses, to fortify our eyesight, since it is necessary to have good eyesight, a good sense of smell, touch, hearing, and taste, etc.

We must remain in this posture for some time, while intensifying our petition to our Divine Mother Kundalini, begging her, beseeching her to help us to attain, with the help of her divine spouse, the benefit, the healing, the faculty, the disintegration of any defect, etc., that we need.

Well, after some time with this posture, after having supplicated to the Divine Mother to bring you the Third Logos and after having totally identified yourself as being one with him so that he

---

19 (Sanskrit) From viparita, "opposite, upside down, reverse, contrary" + karani, "making, doing, form." Mudra "mystic seal."

may heal you or may awaken a particular faculty, etc., you finish the exercise.

Understand that before anything else, we must go to the practical aspect, since these exercises are also effective for the awakening of our chakras, and as I have already stated, through them the Gnostic arhat can enter the path of the awakening of consciousness. You already know the dance of the dervishes, the Viparitakarani Mudra, and the posture of the cross; remember that with our imagination we must open the sick organ by imperatively commanding it:

> **Open Sesame!**
> **Open Sesame!**
> **Open Sesame!**

Comprehend that in each rite-exercise we must beseech our Divine Mother Kundalini so that she can plead to the Holy Spirit in her sacred language. Thus he can assist us and heal us of this or that sickness, according with the necessities we each have, etc. Some will ask for healing, others for the awakening of this or that power, others for the annihilation of this or that defect, etc.

Again, these rites are not merely physical aerobics, but six methods of prayer. It
is a distinct system of healing and rejuvenation through prayer.

The lamas practice these six rites on a
prayer mat; it can be a mat or a carpet or
whatever we want to call it. There are so
many words and each country has many
names in order to name objects or things,
and it is clear that one is forced to use
different terms so that people may understand.

Naturally, with much patience, slowly,
we have to become accustomed to these
exercises. The day will arrive when we will
perform them easily. These are not meant
to be done all at once, no! We must condition our organism slowly, little by little,
in order to perform these exercises better
until they are performed correctly. As far
as conditioning the body is concerned,
some may take days, others weeks, other
months, others years.

These rite-exercises are not for citizens of a particular country either. They
are for all the Gnostic citizens of the
world. I do not understand why people
are bottled up within that which is called
"patriotism." They do not understand

that "my country" and "your country"
are the same country. People have divided
the Earth into parcels and more parcels
and have placed a flag on each parcel, and
chiseled a few statues for their heroes;
they have filled the frontiers with savage
hordes who are armed to the teeth, etc.
Regrettably, this is what they call "my
country." It is very sad that the Earth is
divided into many parcels. The day on
which the Earth will have to change will
arrive. Unfortunately, such a change on
this planet is very difficult. Thus, only
after the great cataclysm will this planet
be converted into one great country...
Nevertheless, now let us limit ourselves to
the exercises that I am teaching you.

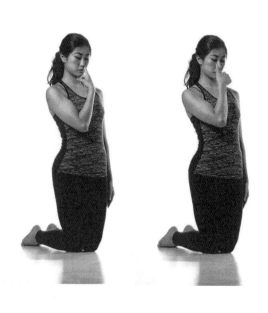

Third Rite

Now, kneel on the floor towards the east, that is, place yourself on your knees, facing where the sun rises, and bow your head a little: only a little, not too much... afterwards you must perform three pranayamas[20] as follows:

PRANAYAMA

Shut your left nostril by placing the index finger of your right hand on it, then inhale air through the right nostril. After the inhalation, close both nostrils with the index finger and the thumb. Hold your breath for a few seconds, then uncover only your left nostril and exhale all the air through it. Now keep the right nostril shut with your thumb on it while inhaling the air through the opened left nostril, then press both nostrils again with the thumb and index finger. Repeat this exercise two more times until you complete three inhalations and three exhalations through each nostril; under-

---

20 Sanskrit for "restraint [ayama] of energy, life force [prana]") A type of breathing exercise which transforms the life force (sexual energy) of the practitioner. See the glossary.

stand that these three inhalations and exhalations are equivalent to three complete pranayamas.

Remember to use only the index finger and the thumb exclusively from the right hand, and that is it. You close one nostril with one finger while inhaling through the opposite nostril, then you close both, and uncover the opposite nostril, etc. It is a back and forth kind of play that you perform from one nostril to the other—that is, when you close one, you uncover the other and vice versa.

Once you have finished your pranayamas, lower your head again and enter into prayer to the Divine Mother Kundalini Shakti, beseeching your Devi Kundalini for what you need, etc.

Now, while in the kneeling position, incline your body back, making an acute angle with it while keeping the kneeling position. Your arms must be kept straight touching the body lengthwise. Incline your body back as far as you can and keep that position for few seconds, while begging, beseeching, imploring to the blessed Mother Kundalini, to intercede for you before the most sacred Holy Spirit so that the benefit you are requesting, whether

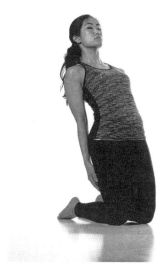

for healing or any other purpose, can be granted.

This exercise is performed in a considerably short time because it is strong or difficult to execute, yet it is very good in order to make the body more agile and to burn some toxins. What is important is to perform it as best we can.

Remember very well that in each exercise, it is necessary to beg, to intensely beseech, to even cry if necessary, in order for our Divine Mother to call upon the

Third Logos in order to heal any given sick organ for us.

Remember that she is the mediator, the one who can invoke the Logos who is her divine spouse, the most sacred Holy Spirit—Shiva,[21] as he is called in the East, the arch-hierophant, the arch-magi, the first begotten of creation, the swan of living plumage, the white dove, the immortal Hiram Abiff,[22] the secret master, whom in the past we all committed the error of murdering. Yes, we murdered him when we committed the original sin.[23] This is why we need to resurrect him from among the dead, and exclaim with all the forces of our heart: *The King is dead; long live the King!*

21 See glossary.
22 A biblical personage; a skillful builder and architect whom King Solomon procured from Tyre for the purpose of supervising the construction of the Temple. According to the Masonic story, Hiram Abiff was murdered by three traitors who were subsequently found by twenty-seven Master Masons.
23 Fornication: the orgasm. See glossary.

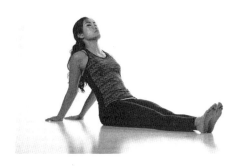

Fourth Rite

Now perform the following position: sit on the floor, place your hands on the floor behind you and stretch your legs so that the trunk of your body is inclined back somewhat and is resting on your hands. Place your heels together, yet with the feet opened like a fan, and your head and eyes looking forward.

Here, we once again make our petition, our supplication, with much faith and devotion for our Divine Mother.

Now, in order to execute the following exercise, let us bend our legs a little until the soles of our feet are placed on the floor. Then we must elevate our but-

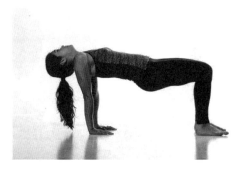

tocks and our belly or abdomen, so that our body is in the position of a table; our knees, abdomen and face must form a straight, horizontal line.

Our face must be looking up, towards the ceiling of the house. The body must be supported by the hands and the feet, thus forming, as I already stated, a human table.

While in this position, we must intensify our imploration and supplication to our blessed Mother Devi Kundalini, asking her to invoke her divine husband, the most sacred Holy Spirit, so that he can come and execute the cure we need. This has been explained to you several times, but it is good to insist upon it so that you do not forget that these rites are not just something physical; they are something different. Each exercise needs imploration and supplication in order to be complete. Understand that exercise and supplication must be equilibrated.

Repeat the Pranayama

Before studying the rite-exercise called Mayurasana, let us now repeat exercise four, but here it will be number eight. So, it is necessary to perform again three pranayamas. I repeat, these are already explained in exercise four.

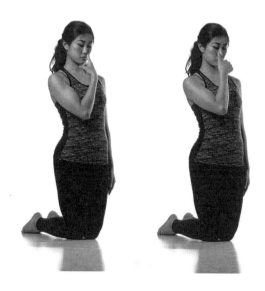

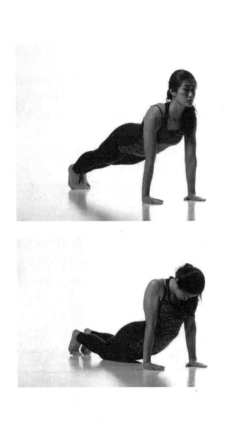

Fifth Rite

Then, after having performed the three pranayamas, we place our body in the position of a lizard; this is why Mayurasana is also called the posture of the lizard.

Many people practice the lizard posture specifically to eliminate their bulging abdomen, in other words, what we call the belly, or that horribly inflated and unhealthy abdomen filled with fat.

The ninth exercise is performed by executing motion between two positions:

FIRST POSITION: hold the body like a lizard as follows: hold your body up with straight arms by placing the palms of your hands on the floor; stretch your legs back and straight, and sustain the rest of your body on your feet, your tiptoes, with your face looking forward. The back, neck, buttocks, legs, and heels must maintain a straight line, just like a lizard.

SECOND POSITION: while keeping your arms and legs straight, lower your head, tuck it to your chest as much as you can, and lower the knees, legs, and abdomen.

Thereafter, repeat this movement: downwards, upwards, downwards, upwards, etc.

Here, we implore to our Divine Mother to activate all of our chakras.

When lowering the head and tucking it below the chest as much as we can, we must also lower the knees, legs, and abdomen together, without moving the hands and feet from their initial position, then we rise to the position of the ninth exercise, then we lower to the position of the tenth exercise, up and down, up and down, etc...

From the tenth position of the lizard, where we have our head well tucked under our chest, without moving our hands and keeping our arms in a straight position and keeping our head well tucked underneath our chest as much as we can, with straight legs, we advance few short steps forward, until our body becomes a human arch.

Resting on our hands and feet and with the head well-tucked to our chest, forming a perfect human arc, we must enter into prayer, asking, begging, beseeching, as I have already taught you, to our Divine Mother for what we most need. Underneath your body cars and car-

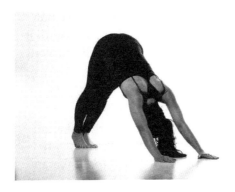

riages can pass, since it is forming a type of human arch.

Now, after having prayed for a while in the arch position, we bend our knees a little in order to lower our body, and then lift our hands from the floor; we get up, in other words. We stand straight up on our feet, thus finishing with the exercise.

Remember that with this position of the human arc, just as we have shown it, we make the blood to rush towards the head and the lymph to cleanse and irrigate all the cranial zones.

All of these are very special exercises that help to terminate with the belly or paunch; I do not know why people love to maintain their bulging stomachs filled with fat: ironically they call it "the curve of happiness." We must never have our stomach filled with fat. Understand that with this exercise, we say goodbye to our potbelly.

Viparitakarani Mudra

Now let us learn the Viparitakarani Mudra in a special manner in order to rejuvenate the body. The Viparitakarani Mudra as an twelfth exercise is as follows: Lie down on your back on the floor with your buttocks and legs against a wall, that is, raise your legs and place them in a vertical position against a wall. For this posture place your buttocks and legs very close to the wall while your lower and upper back rests on the floor; hands and arms rest on the floor parallel to the body.

This exercise is special in order to perform a great work that can only be executed by the most sacred Holy Spirit, within our organism.

In our brain we have a moon that makes us the most lunar beings in this world; thus, for the reason that the moon is in our brain, our actions are negative and lunar. On the other hand, we have a marvelous sun in the umbilical region (solar plexus). Thus, from the time we exited paradise, the luminous sun that was in the brain was transferred to the umbilical region (solar plexus) and the cold moon went up to the brain.

Therefore, understanding that we have this alteration in our organism, while we lie down in that position, we beg to the most sacred Holy Spirit to execute a transplantation within us: that is, to transfer the moon from our brain and to settle it in our umbilical region, and to simultaneously transfer the luminous sun from our umbilical region (solar plexus) and to settle it in our brain.

It is clear that it is essential to practice the Viparitakarani Mudra incessantly, constantly, permanently, just as we are showing it, and to beg, plead, beseech the Holy Spirit to grant us the grace of making this mutation, that is, to place the moon that we have in our brain in our umbilical region and to transfer the sun that we have in our umbilical region to our brain.

This is a labor that only the Third Logos can perform, and the Viparitakarani Mudra is the precise, necessary posture for it. We must profoundly implore and beseech, while concentrating on the Third Logos, so that he may come and perform the transplantation of the moon to the umbilical region and the sun to the brain.

This Viparitakarani Mudra is a truly marvelous rite in order to attain the rejuvenation of the physical body. To reconquer everlasting youth is urgent and necessary, since the body should remain young and vigorous in any initiate who marches upon the path of the razor's edge.

Whosoever achieves the performance of the Viparitakarani Mudra straight for three hours will defeat death and will reconquer everlasting youth. Nevertheless, we must begin by performing for no more than five minutes at a time, and thereafter we increase the time gradually, slowly, patiently; for instance, increase it by one minute daily.

For those who aspire for the rejuvenation of their body and for the healing of all sickness, here we give them this marvelous formula: the Viparitakarani Mudra. Understood?

So, in the Viparitakarani Mudra we ask the Third Logos for the rejuvenation of our physical organism or to heal us from any malady or sickness, to replace the old cells for new cells, etc. Start with five minutes and add progressively one minute every day until reaching the maximum of three hours. It is evident that in order to achieve the three hours, a long time is necessary, maybe several years of constant practice, yet those years of constant practice are equivalent to defeating death by means of the famous Viparitakarani Mudra.

> "The esoteric Viparitakarani teaches scientifically how the Hindu yogi, instead of ejaculating the semen, raises it slowly through concentration in such a way that a man and woman can eliminate the animal ego while united sexually. The esoteric Viparitakarani teaches how, through concentration, the "yogi slowly raises the semen, in such a way that man and woman can attain Vajroli." As stated in the Viparitakarani: "This practice is the most excellent one, the cause of liberation for the yogi; this practice brings health to a yogi and grants

him perfection." —Samael Aun Weor, *The Mystery of the Golden Blossom*

Sixth Rite

We are now entering into the study of
the sixth rite that is precisely the Vajroli
Mudra, which is the rite related with the
transmutation of the sexual energy, which
is the finest type of energy that is gener-
ated by the physical organism; it is, better
said, the subtlest force with which the
human body works.

The human vehicle has certain very
fine channels through which the sexual
energy circulates; this energy cannot cir-
culate through other channels, because
when the sexual energy bursts into other
channels, it is clear that a catastrophe
takes place. The sexual energy is a wonderful, explosive force that we must learn
how to direct wisely, if we truly want the
inner realization of the Being.

Indubitably, the Vajroli Mudra is a
very special rite for bachelors and bachelorettes, even though it can also aid
married people. Specifically, we can say
that with the Vajroli Mudra the bachelors

and bachelorettes have a fundamental system in order to sustain themselves in Brahmacharya[24]—that is, in chastity.[25]

Men and women who do not have a spouse must sustain themselves in Brahmacharya—of course, until the day in which the bachelor acquires his priestess and the bachelorette her husband.

Many bachelors and bachelorettes would like to fulfill their sexual functions here, there, and everywhere with different partners—that is, to fornicate[26]—yet, that is prohibited for the aspirants to the adepthood. Bachelors and bachelorettes who truly aspire to reach adepthood cannot mix sexually with different partners, because by doing so they violate the law—that is, they break the sixth commandment of the law of God.[27]

Celibates must firmly maintain themselves in Brahmacharya until their spouse arrives to them, and it is not possible for

---

24 Sexual continence: ie. no orgasm. See glossary.
25 Sexual purity. This is not repression or abstinence from sex, but is instead sexual transmutation. See glossary.
26 Fornication is to waste sexual energy, especially through orgasm. See glossary.
27 "Thou shalt not fornicate (orgasm)." See Numbers 21 in the Bible.

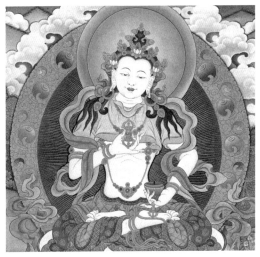

Vajrapani, symbol of the power of all bud-
dhas. In his hands are the vajra (masculine sexual
power) and bell (feminine sexual power).

them to maintain their Brahmacharya if
they do not know how to transmute their
sexual energy.

Whosoever wants to learn how to
transmute the sexual energy must know
in depth the Vajroli Mudra, since if
they do not know it, they do not know,
because they do not have the science for
sexual transmutation.[28]

---

28 Sexual transmutation is also called tantra,
    alchemy, karezza, coitus interruptus, etc.

Vajroli Mudra has—among other things—an advantage especially for bachelors, in spite of being unmarried, to preserve their sexual potency—that is, not to lose their virility. Normally, an organ that is not used becomes atrophied. If one ceases to use one hand, then that hand becomes atrophied. If one ceases to use a foot, then that foot does not work anymore. Likewise, if one ceases to use one's creative organs, then they simply become atrophied and the man becomes impotent; then, such a man is already marching with a deficiency.

Fortunately, with the Vajroli Mudra bachelors can preserve their sexual potency for their entire life. However, I am not saying, and I clarify this, that an individual can create the superior existential bodies[29] of the Being with the Vajroli Mudra; no! I am not making these types of affirmations. Neither am I stating that with the Vajroli Mudra one can attain the inner realization of the Being. Whosoever wants to attain inner realization has to work in the forge of the Cyclops[30]—this is clear. It

29 The solar astral, mental, and causal bodies. For more on this, read *The Narrow Way* by Samael Aun Weor.

30 Sex between husband and wife.

so happens that with the Vajroli Mudra
one is only working with a single force;
in the case of the man, he works with
the masculine force, and in the case of
the woman, with the feminine force, and
nothing else. In order to create the superior existential bodies of the Being, something more is necessary; it is required to
work with the three forces of nature and
the cosmos: the masculine force (in the
man), the feminine force (in the woman),
and the neutral force (that in the sexual
act conciliates the masculine and feminine). As I have already stated, the masculine force is the Holy Affirmation, the
feminine force is the Holy Negation, and
the neutral force is the Holy Conciliation.
It is clear that in order for creation to
occur the three forces are necessary; this is
why the Sahaja Maithuna[31] is indispensable in order to create the superior existential bodies of the Being.

Common and ordinary people do not
have the astral, mental, and causal bodies
because such bodies have to be created,
and they can only be created by means
of the Sahaja Maithuna or Sexual Magic.
Nevertheless, I repeat, the Vajroli Mudra

---

31 Sanskrit, "original sexual act." See glossary.

serves the bachelors since they do not
have wife, and bachelorettes since they do
not have a husband, and it also helps the
couples that are working with the Sahaja
Maithuna, because it helps them to sublimate and transmute their sexual energy.
Therefore, the Vajroli Mudra is very useful for bachelors and bachelorettes and
for married couples. Well, now after this
explanation, I am going to teach the technique of the Vajroli Mudra.

Standing in a steady position, looking
forward, place your hands on your waist
with your thumbs towards your lower
back—thus making with your arms the
shape of a jar's handles—then inhale air
until totally filling the lungs. Next, put
the palms of your hands on top of your
thighs and incline your body forward—
not towards the sides nor backwards,
but forward as when one is assuming a
reclining position or making a profound
prostration—thus, continue lowering the
palms of your hands little by little until
reaching your knees. As you bend, simultaneously you must exhale the air, so that
when you are already touching your knees
your lungs are completely empty of air.

Once in the leaning position, we are
prepared to continue the sequence of the
exercise. Here, still, we have not inhaled
the air: our lungs are completely empty.
Now, we continue the exercise by raising
the hands in the direction of the creative
organs—yet, we must not fill the lungs
with air—now we perform a massage on
the belly at the level of the prostate /
uterus, so that the vibration reaches the
prostate or uterus and the transmutation of the sexual energy is performed; we
must perform a massage not only on level
of the prostate or uterus, but we must
also perform a massage with firmness
upon the sexual organs. Then, as soon as
we perform the massage over the creative
organs, we must slowly raise the body to
an upright position; thus, we straighten
the body while our feet remain united
and firm on the floor. Now, with the body
straight, we place the hands on the waist,
thus with the arms making again the
shape of a jar's handles.

Once we have performed the massage and have placed the hands on the
waist, we inhale until filling our lungs
with air, and sublimate the sexual energy
to the brain through the channels Ida

and Pingala.[32] Then, we exhale slowly and repeat the same procedure three times.

Regarding the massages at the level of the prostate / uterus and the sexual organs, there are three types:

- a) Gentle massage upon the abdomen at the level of the prostate / uterus and creative organs.

- b) Moderate massage upon the region of the prostate / uterus and creative organs.

- c) Strong massage upon the region of the prostate / uterus and creative organs.

It is obvious that for men a strong massage on the area of the prostate and sexual organs produces the erection of the phallus; this is clearly how it is. This is why the third type of massage is advisable for bachelors. Thus, when the phallus is erected, the transmutation of the semen into energy is produced, which one raises to the brain.

Regarding married men, the first or second types of massages are convenient for them, nothing else; rather, the first

---

32 Two subtle channels of energy that intertwine along the spine.

type is more than enough since they have
a wife and of course they bring the phallus to a complete erection by means of the
Sahaja Maithuna.

So, here I have taught you what in the
East they call Vajroli Mudra.

In the case of women, the Vajroli
Mudra is the same, with the difference
that women must perform the massages
over their left and right ovaries and over
their feminine organs—to be more precise,
over the vagina, the yoni. This is how the
transmutation of the sexual energy takes
place in women.

The same applies to the married
woman, although she does not need a
strong massage, only a soft one; bachelorettes need a little stronger massage
in order to produce the transmutation of
their sexual energy; it is necessary that the
energy raises to the brain.

Therefore, it is necessary to have a
great force of willpower during the Vajroli
Mudra. No lustful thought must cross
the mind of the student. It is necessary to
control the senses. It is necessary to sub-
jugate the mind.

When one practices the Vajroli
Mudra, one needs to be concentrated on

the Divine Mother Kundalini, or on the Third Logos. If one is concentrated exclusively on the sexual organs and forgets the Divine Mother and the Third Logos, then one does not sublimate the sexual energy, and one goes against the cosmic law.

Moreover, take into account that if the human being does not have enough purity in his thoughts, he can degenerate himself and become a masturbator. For the impure and masturbators will be the abyss and the second death,[33] "where only weeping and gnashing of teeth are heard."[34]

Therefore, the Vajroli Mudra is for completely chaste men and women who truly are willing to follow the path of absolute chastity.

The strong—very strong—Vajroli Mudra can only be practiced once a day,

---

33 The Second Death is the complete dissolution of the ego (karma, defects, sins) in the infernal regions of nature, which after unimaginable quantities of suffering, proportional to the density of the psyche, in the end purifies the Essence (consciousness) so that it may try again to perfect itself and reach the union with the Being. To learn about it, read books by Samael Aun Weor such as *The Aquarian Message* or *Beyond Death*.

34 Matthew 8:12, 13:42, 13:50, etc.

and for this it is necessary for the individual to be very serious and respectful of their body; this for bachelors and bachelorettes, since a married man does not need to practice a strong Vajroli, because he attains erection with his priestess wife. Likewise, a woman who has a husband does not need to practice strong Vajroli, because she transmutes her energies with her husband. Therefore, married couples must perform extremely soft massages during the practices of Vajroli; what one is aiming is to elevate that subtle and delicate creative energy to the brain.

In the case of a married man, it is enough, as I already stated, for a slight massage on region of the prostate and sexual organs; likewise for the married woman, a slight massage on the region of the ovaries and the uterus. A very subtle and smooth massage does no harm in any way. Thus it is possible to practice a slight massage whenever we work with the six rites taught in this book, without the slightest damage. Thus, this is how the sexual energy is constantly, incessantly sublimated, and used for our regeneration.

I am therefore, speaking in a very clear manner so that you can understand me.

This system as I have taught it to you here is the Tibetan system.

I repeat that it is necessary to perform it with purity and without lust, nor evil, passional thoughts; otherwise, if the students misuse these teachings, then the sword's edge turns against them and they can tumble into the abyss.

So, I believe that the Gnostic brothers and sisters have understood the purpose of the Vajroli Mudra. Again, I am not tired of repeating that this is the most practical and precise system of sexual transmutation for bachelors and bachelorettes.

After teaching the practice of Vajroli Mudra, I must state the following: The fatal antithesis of the Vajroli Mudra is the horrifying, impure, and abominable vice of masturbation. Those who practice masturbation sink into the abyss in order to suffer the second death, because of the crime of having had profaned their body, because of having—with their perverted deeds—insulted and profaned the Holy Spirit, the Third Logos.

Therefore, be very careful, brothers and sisters who practice the Vajroli Mudra, of not falling into the abominable and repugnant vice of masturbation. The Vajroli Mudra is something very holy, very sacred; a tremendous chastity, a great sanctity, an enormous love to the very sacred Holy Spirit and the Divine Mother Kundalini are required in order to practice it.

I must also clarify that I am not stating here that with the Vajroli Mudra one is going to awaken the Kundalini, or that one can create the superior existential bodies of the Being; no! The Vajroli Mudra only transmutes the semen[35] into energy, and that is all.

It is already clear that in order to awaken the Kundalini it is necessary to have the cooperation of the three forces of nature and the cosmos, as we already stated, but it is worthwhile to remember it once again so that you may record it very well in your minds. The first force is the Holy Affirmation, the second force is the Holy Negation, and the third force is the Holy Conciliation; the lat-

---

35 The word semen literally means "seed," which is within women and men.

ter unites and conciliates the other two. Therefore, the Kundalini can only be developed by means of Sexual Magic, Sahaja Maithuna—in other words, with the cooperation of the three forces. The man has the positive force, the woman has the negative force, and the Holy Spirit conciliates them; thus, the Divine Princess Kundalini awakens with the fusion of the three forces.

The superior existential bodies of the Being cannot be created with a solitary force. The man has one force: this is the Holy Affirmation. The woman only has the negative force: this is, the Holy Negation. It is only possible to perform creation with the union of the three forces: the positive or masculine, the negative or feminine, and the neutral that coordinates and mixes both.

Transmutation[36] is always indispensable, since it is an organic and fundamental necessity.

---

36 To change from one substance or form to another. A term from alchemy, whose entire science is focused on the change of the impure into the pure. "No one can Self-realize without transmutation." —Samael Aun Weor, *Tarot and Kabbalah*

Well, it was necessary to have spoken clearly on this aspect, since the Vajroli Mudra—which is a marvelous system for transmutation for bachelors and bachelorettes—is practiced, for instance, in India, in Tibet, and in that monastery named "the Spring of Eternal Youth."

So, the objective of this system is to elevate the creative energy to the brain. In other words, this is how we seminally nourish the brain and this is how we cerebrally nourish the semen.

Editor's Epilogue: Vajroli Mudra

The term Vajroli Mudra comes from Sanskrit vajra, "thunderbolt, lightning, diamond, adamantine, phallus" and mudra, "mystical seal." In various Asian traditions, the term refers to practices in Hindu and Tibetan Yogas, albeit with an incredible amount of variation and even opposing uses. Some vajroli techniques (such as the one taught by Samael Aun Weor) are positive and valuable, but most of those known to the public are degenerated, ranging from useless to dangerous. Readers may also be surprised to discover that the Vajroli Mudra technique taught

by Samael Aun Weor does not correspond
to the versions known by aficionados of
Eastern mysticism. It is in the interest of
the student to meditate on the disparity,
and consider well how reliable and sincere
a source of knowledge the general public
(or even the so-called experts in Tantra)
may be, especially those who make their
living from their "expertise." One such
popular technique, taught widely in many
different schools of Tantra, is briefly
described by Samael Aun Weor:

> "It causes us great horror to know
> that the tenebrous black magicians
> of the Drukpa clan (those who are
> dedicated to the fatal and horrible
> black tantra) ejaculate the seminal
> liquor during their practices of
> black magic. These black magicians
> have a fatal technique that enables
> them to reabsorb the spilled semen.
> Such a technique is known as black
> vajroli. This practice is completely
> negative; therefore we do not even
> want to explain the procedure. We
> know that there exist many people
> with very weak mentalities, who
> could easily be led into practicing
> such horrible black tantra. Karma

would then fatally fall upon us. The spilled semen is mixed with feminine "verya" (feminine semen) and afterwards it is re-absorbed. Thus, it is horribly recharged with atoms of the secret enemy. These are satanic atoms that are collected from the atomic infernos of the human being. The inevitable result of this black tantra is the descent of the serpent towards the atomic abyss of Nature. This is how the human personality ends. It is definitely disconnected from its Divine Spirit. The human being is then transformed into a demon. "The Arcanum A.Z.F. (Oordhvarata) was practiced within the ashrams of ancient India. At that time, yogis were prepared for sexual magic with the white vajroli. Unfortunately, the brothers and sisters of the temple committed scandalous acts, which discredited sexual magic. The Gurujis then pulled the curtains of esotericism shut, and the Arcanum A.Z.F. was forbidden." —Samael Aun Weor, *The Yellow Book*

Obviously, the Vajroli Mudra technique taught in this book belongs to the Tantra of chastity and is directly opposed to the Vajrolis taught in the Tantric schools of fornication, whether in the East or the West, which are very popular and widespread in these dark times.

To learn more about sexual transmutation, we recommend the book *The Perfect Matrimony* by Samael Aun Weor.

Glossary

Astral: This term is derived from "pertaining to or proceeding from the stars," but in the esoteric knowledge it refers to the emotional aspect of the fifth dimension, which in Hebrew is called Hod.

Astral Body: The body utilized by the consciousness in the fifth dimension, the world of dreams. This body is related to the emotional center and to the sephirah Hod.

"...the astral body is material, and it is a dense organism like the physical body. The fact that matter, in its last synthesis, is reduced to energy, does not deny its existence once in that state. If we cannot see it with our sense of sight, it is because it belongs to the fifth dimension. Our physical eyes will not serve for seeing the astral plane until we make them suitable for this purpose or until we place ourselves into the astral plane with our physical body. Thus, the astral organism is as dense as the physical organism, yet it belongs to another department of the kingdom. The astral body is much more sensitive than the physical body. The astral organism is like a duplicate of the physical organism. As the physical body has to be nourished with food related to its nature, so does the astral body. The occultist utilizes the astral body for his studies and for his great investigations, because that body is advantageously arranged over the physical body. Time and distance do not exist for the astral body, and what one learns through it remains immediately recorded within the consciousness of the Being, forever." —Samael Aun Weor, *The Revolution of Beelzebub*

"During the hours of sleep all human beings travel in the [lunar] astral body, but they disgracefully live in the astral plane with the consciousness asleep. They are sleeping wanderers." —Samael Aun Weor, *The Aquarian Message*

What is commonly called the astral body is not the true astral body, it is rather the lunar protoplasmatic body, also known as the kama rupa (Sanskrit, "body of desires") or "dream body" (Tibetan rmi-lam-gyi lus). The true astral body is solar (being superior to lunar nature) and must be created, as the Master Jesus indicated in the Gospel of John 3:5-6,

"Except a man be born of water and of the Spirit, he cannot enter into the kingdom of God. That which is born of the flesh is flesh; and that which is born of the Spirit is spirit."

The solar astral body is created as a result of the third initiation of major mysteries (serpents of fire), and is perfected in the third serpent of light.

"Really, only those who have worked with the maithuna (white tantra) for many years can possess the astral body." - Samael Aun Weor, *The Elimination of Satan's Tail*

"THE [LUNAR] ASTRAL BODY.—A sheath of radiant, fluidic atmosphere that envelops the physical form and is seen by the third eye. It registers our passions and desires and is a remnant of the past." —M, *The Dayspring of Youth*

"We have the longing of visiting or entering the sephirothic regions of space. One thing is to grasp a sephirah and another thing is to enter it. Obviously, the sephiroth are atomic, and we, the Gnostics, must enter the Tree of Life. We must know that there are many sephirothic regions in space; to enter them is marvelous. How are we going to enter the Kabbalistic region of Hod if we do not have a psychological body? There are psychological projections (astral projections). The diverse psychological aggregates can, at any given moment, integrate themselves in order to enter the sephirah Hod (astral world, or first heaven). But that would only be a subjective entrance; that would not have objectivity such as when the second body (solar astral body) has been created. This body has to be created in order to handle the emotions of this region. What type of emotions am I referring to? I am referring to superior emotions. The inferior emotions are an obstacle for experiencing what is reality (God), and for the psychological development of the Being. If we want to be born again, to create a second body, in order to enter into the sephirothic region of Hod (the king-dom of heaven), then it is obvious that we should not torpidly waste our energies by letting ourselves be pulled in by negative emotions, such as violence, hatred, jealousy, pride, etc." —Samael Aun Weor, *Alcyone and Negative Emotions*

Brahmacharya: Brahmacharya is a Sanskrit word (ब्रह्मचर्य) composed from Brahma, the Creative Force, God; and charya, "to be followed; observance or restraint."

"Brahmacharya literally means Achara or conduct that leads to the realization of Brahman or one's own Self. It means the control of semen [the sexual seed, which is in men and women], the study of the Vedas (scriptures) and contemplation on God. The technical meaning of Brahmacharya is self-restraint, particularly mastery of perfect control over the sexual organ or freedom from lust in thought, word and deed." - Swami Sivananda

Brahamcharya is sexual purity, meaning that the orgasm is avoided, forbidden. One renounces the low, animal pleasure of the orgasm in order to gain the higher, spiritual bliss of the soul:

"Ejaculation of semen [orgasm] brings death, preserving it within brings life. Therefore, one should make sure to retain the semen within. One is born and dies through semen; in this there is no doubt. Knowing this, the Yogi must always preserve his semen. When the precious jewel of semen is mastered, anything on earth can be mastered. Through the grace of its preservation, one becomes as great as me [Shiva]. The use of semen determines the happiness or pain of all beings living in the world, who are deluded [by desire] and are subject to death and decay."
—Siva Samhita

Brahmacharya is not merely a physical restraint: it is also mental.

"The technical meaning of Brahmacharya is self-restraint, particularly mastery of perfect control over the sexual organ or freedom from lust in thought, word and deed. Strict abstinence is not merely from sexual intercourse, but also from auto-erotic manifestations, from homosexual acts and from all perverse sexual practices. It must further involve a permanent abstention from indulgence in erotic imagination and voluptuous reverie. All sorts of sex anomalies and evil habits of various sorts like masturbation and sodomy must be completely eradicated. They bring about a total breakdown of the nervous system and immense misery.

"Brahmacharya is purity in thought, word and deed... Brahmacharya is absolute freedom from sexual desires and thoughts. A real Brahmachari will not feel any difference in touching a woman, a piece of paper or a block of wood. Brahmacharya is meant for both men and women. Bhishma, Hanuman, Lakshman, Mira Bai, Sulabha and Gargi were all established in Brahmacharya.

"Mere control of the animal passion will not constitute Brahmacharya. This is incomplete Brahmacharya. You must control all the organs— the ears that want to hear lustful stories, the lustful eye that wants to see objects that excite passion, the tongue that wants to taste exciting things and the skin that wants to touch exciting objects.

"To look lustfully is adultery of the eyes; to hear anything that excites passion is adultery of the ears; to speak anything that excites passion is adultery of the tongue." - Swami Sivananda

Many great teachers of Yoga and Hinduism maintained a public image of celibacy but privately taught and practiced Tantra. Notable examples include Swami Sivananda and Ramakrishna.

Some teachers renounced the higher path of Tantra, such as Paramahansa Yogananda. His teachers were married.

As such, there are two primary modes of Brahamacharya:

Lunar: celibacy and sexual repression, in which the sexual impulse is merely denied, not transformed.

Solar: celibacy with transmutation. Such a stage can occur before or after marriage (such as after the death of a spouse), or if the work of matrimony is already complete (such as St. Paul).

Centers, Seven: The human being has seven centers of psychological activity. The first five are the Intellectual, Emotional, Motor, Instinctive, and Sexual Centers. However, through inner development one learns how to utilize the Superior Emotional and Superior Intellectual Centers. Most people do not use these two at all.

Chakra: (Sanskrit) Literally, "wheel." The chakras are subtle centers of energetic transformation. There are hundreds of chakras in our multi-dimensional physiology.

"The chakras are points of connection through which the divine energy circulates from one to another vehicle of the human being." - Samael Aun Weor, *Aztec Christic Magic*

Chastity: Although modern usage has rendered the term chastity virtually meaningless to most people, its original meaning and usage clearly indicate "moral purity" upon the basis of "sexual purity." Contemporary usage implies "repression" or "abstinence," which have nothing to do with real chastity. True chastity is a rejection of impure sexuality. True chastity is pure sexuality, or the activity of sex in harmony with our true nature, as explained in the secret doctrine. Properly used, the word chastity refers to sexual fidelity or honor.

"The generative energy, which, when we are loose, dissipates and makes us unclean, when we are continent invigorates and inspires us. Chastity is the flowering of man; and what are called Genius, Heroism, Holiness, and the like, are but various fruits which succeed it." —Henry David Thoreau, *Walden*

Consciousness: "Wherever there is life, there is consciousness. Consciousness is inherent to life as humidity is inherent to water." —Samael Aun Weor, *Sexology, the Basis of Endocrinology and Criminology*

From various dictionaries: 1. The state of being conscious; knowledge of one's own existence, condition, sensations, mental operations, acts, etc. 2. Immediate knowledge or perception of the presence of any object, state, or sensation. 3. An alert cognitive state in which you are aware of yourself and your situation. In universal Gnosticism, the range of potential consciousness is allegorized in the Ladder of Jacob, upon which the angels ascend and descend. Thus there are higher and lower levels of consciousness, from the level of demons at the bottom, to highly realized angels in the heights.

"It is vital to understand and develop the conviction that consciousness has the potential to increase to an infinite degree." —The 14th Dalai Lama

"Light and consciousness are two phenomena of the same thing; to a lesser degree of consciousness, corresponds a lesser degree of light; to a greater degree of consciousness, a greater degree of light." —Samael Aun Weor, *The Esoteric Treatise of Hermetic Astrology*

Divine Mother: The feminine, receptive force through which creation occurs, symbolized in many religions by figures such as Isis, Mary, Maya, Tara, Isobertha, Rhea, Cybele, Gaea, etc. The formless-force-matter symbolizing Nature, whose conception and childbirth reveals the fertility of Nature. In Hebrew, Eloah, the feminine counterpart of El, whose union produces Elohim.

"Among the Aztecs, she was known as Tonantzin, among the Greeks as chaste Diana. In Egypt she was Isis, the Divine Mother, whose veil no mortal has lifted. There is no doubt at all that esoteric Christianity has never forsaken the worship of the Divine Mother Kundalini. Obviously she is Marah, or better said, RAM-IO, MARY. What orthodox religions did not specify, at least with regard to the exoteric or public circle, is the aspect of Isis in her individual human form. Clearly, it was taught only in secret to the Initiates that this Divine Mother exists individually within each human being. It cannot be emphasized enough that Mother-God, Rhea, Cybele, Adonia, or whatever we wish to call her, is a variant of our own individual Being in the here and now. Stated explicitly, each of us has

our own particular, individual Divine Mother."
—Samael Aun Weor, *The Great Rebellion*

"Devi Kundalini, the Consecrated Queen of
Shiva, our personal Divine Cosmic Individual
Mother, assumes five transcendental mystic
aspects in every creature, which we must enu-
merate:

1. The unmanifested Prakriti

2. The chaste Diana, Isis, Tonantzin, Maria or
better said Ram-Io

3. The terrible Hecate, Persephone, Coatlicue,
queen of the infernos and death; terror of love
and law

4. The special individual Mother Nature, creator
and architect of our physical organism

5. The Elemental Enchantress to whom we owe
every vital impulse, every instinct." —Samael
Aun Weor, *The Mystery of the Golden Blossom*

Drukpa: (Also known variously as Druk-pa, Dugpa,
Brugpa, Dag dugpa or Dad dugpa) The term
Drukpa comes from from Dzongkha and Tibetan 'brug yul, which means "country of Bhutan,"
and is composed of Druk, "dragon," and pa,
"person." In Asia, the word refers to the people of
Bhutan, a country between India and Tibet.

Drukpa can also refer to a large sect of Buddhism which broke from the Kagyug-pa "the
Ones of the Oral Tradition." They considered
themselves as the heirs of the indian Gurus:
their teaching, which goes back to Vajradhara,
was conveyed through Dakini, from Naropa to
Marpa and then to the ascetic and mystic poet
Milarepa. Later on, Milarepa's disciples founded

new monasteries, and new threads appeared, among which are the Karmapa and the Drukpa. All those schools form the Kagyug-pa order, in spite of episodic internal quarrels and extreme differences in practice. The Drukpa sect is recognized by their ceremonial large red hats, but it should be known that they are not the only "Red Hat" group (the Nyingmas, founded by Padmasambhava, also use red hats). The Drukpas have established a particular worship of the Dorje (Vajra, or thunderbolt, a symbol of the phallus).

Samael Aun Weor wrote repeatedly in many books that the "Drukpas" practice and teach Black Tantra, by means of the expelling of the sexual energy. If we analyze the word, it is clear that he is referring to "Black Dragons," or people who practice Black Tantra. He was not referring to all the people of Bhutan, or all members of the Buddhist Drukpa sect. Such a broad condemnation would be as ridiculous as the one made by all those who condemn all Jews for the crucifixion of Jesus.

"In 1387, with just reason, the Tibetan reformer Tsong Khapa cast every book of Necromancy that he found into flames. As a result, some discontent Lamas formed an alliance with the aboriginal Bhons, and today they form a powerful sect of black magic in the regions of Sikkim, Bhutan, and Nepal, submitting themselves to the most abominable black rites." —Samael Aun Weor, *The Revolution of Beelzebub*

Ego: The multiplicity of contradictory psychological elements that we have inside are in their sum the "ego." Each one is also called "an ego" or an

"I." Every ego is a psychological defect which produces suffering. The ego is three (related to our Three Brains or three centers of psychological processing), seven (capital sins), and legion (in their infinite variations).

"The ego is the root of ignorance and pain." — Samael Aun Weor, *The Esoteric Treatise of Hermetic Astrology*

"The Being and the ego are incompatible. The Being and the ego are like water and oil. They can never be mixed... The annihilation of the psychic aggregates (egos) can be made possible only by radically comprehending our errors through meditation and by the evident Self-reflection of the Being." —Samael Aun Weor, *The Gnostic Bible: The Pistis Sophia Unveiled*

Fornication: Originally, the term fornication was derived from the Indo-European word gwher, whose meanings relate to heat and burning. Fornication means to make the heat (solar fire) of the seed (sexual power) leave the body through voluntary orgasm. Any voluntary orgasm is fornication, whether between a married man and woman, or an unmarried man and woman, or through masturbation, or in any other case; this is explained by Moses: "A man from whom there is a discharge of semen, shall immerse all his flesh in water, and he shall remain unclean until evening. And any garment or any leather [object] which has semen on it, shall be immersed in water, and shall remain unclean until evening. A woman with whom a man cohabits, whereby there was [a discharge of] semen, they shall immerse in water, and they shall remain unclean until evening." —Leviticus 15:16-18

To fornicate is to spill the sexual energy through the orgasm. Those who "deny themselves" restrain the sexual energy, and "walk in the midst of the fire" without being burned. Those who restrain the sexual energy, who renounce the orgasm, remember God in themselves, and do not defile themselves with animal passion, "for the temple of God is holy, which temple ye are."

"Whosoever is born of God doth not commit sin; for his seed remaineth in him: and he cannot sin, because he is born of God." —1 John 3:9

This is why neophytes always took a vow of sexual abstention, so that they could prepare themselves for marriage, in which they would have sexual relations but not release the sexual energy through the orgasm. This is why Paul advised:

"...they that have wives be as though they had none..." —I Corinthians 7:29

"A fornicator is an individual who has intensely accustomed his genital organs to copulate (with orgasm). Yet, if the same individual changes his custom of copulation to the custom of no copulation, then he transforms himself into a chaste person. We have as an example the astonishing case of Mary Magdalene, who was a famous prostitute. Mary Magdalene became the famous Saint Mary Magdalene, the repented prostitute. Mary Magdalene became the chaste disciple of Christ." —Samael Aun Weor, *The Revolution of Beelzebub*

Gnosis: (Greek) Knowledge.

1. The word Gnosis refers to the knowledge we acquire through our own experience, as opposed to knowledge that we are told or believe in. Gnosis - by whatever name in history or culture - is conscious, experiential knowledge, not merely intellectual or conceptual knowledge, belief, or theory. This term is synonymous with the Hebrew "daath" and the Sanskrit "jna."

2. The tradition that embodies the core wisdom or knowledge of humanity.

"Gnosis is the flame from which all religions sprouted, because in its depth Gnosis is religion. The word "religion" comes from the Latin word "religare," which implies "to link the Soul to God"; so Gnosis is the very pure flame from where all religions sprout, because Gnosis is knowledge, Gnosis is wisdom." —Samael Aun Weor, *The Esoteric Path*

"The secret science of the Sufis and of the Whirling Dervishes is within Gnosis. The secret doctrine of Buddhism and of Taoism is within Gnosis. The sacred magic of the Nordics is within Gnosis. The wisdom of Hermes, Buddha, Confucius, Mohammed and Quetzalcoatl, etc., etc., is within Gnosis. Gnosis is the Doctrine of Christ." —Samael Aun Weor, *The Revolution of Beelzebub*

Holy Spirit: The Christian name for the third aspect of the Holy Trinity, or "God." This force has other names in other religions. In Kabbalah, the third sephirah, Binah. In Buddhism, it is related to Nirmanakaya, the "body of formation" through which the inner Buddha works in the world.

"The Holy Spirit is the Fire of Pentecost or the fire of the Holy Spirit called Kundalini by the Hindus, the igneous serpent of our magical powers, Holy Fire symbolized by Gold..." — Samael Aun Weor, *The Perfect Matrimony*

"It has been said in *The Divine Comedy* with complete clarity that the Holy Spirit is the husband of the Divine Mother. Therefore, the Holy Spirit unfolds himself into his wife, into the Shakti of the Hindus. This must be known and understood. Some, when they see that the Third Logos is unfolded into the Divine Mother Kundalini, or Shakti, She that has many names, have believed that the Holy Spirit is feminine, and they have been mistaken. The Holy Spirit is masculine, but when He unfolds Himself into She, then the first ineffable Divine Couple is formed, the Creator Elohim, the Kabir, or Great Priest, the Ruach Elohim, that in accordance to Moses, cultivated the waters in the beginning of the world." —Samael Aun Weor, *Tarot and Kabbalah*

"The Primitive Gnostic Christians worshipped the lamb, the fish and the white dove as symbols of the Holy Spirit." —Samael Aun Weor, *The Perfect Matrimony*

Innermost: "Our real Being is of a universal nature. Our real Being is neither a kind of superior nor inferior "I." Our real Being is impersonal, universal, divine. He transcends every concept of "I," me, myself, ego, etc., etc." —Samael Aun Weor, *The Perfect Matrimony*

Also known as Atman, the Spirit, Chesed, our own individual interior divine Father.

"The Innermost is the ardent flame of Horeb. In accordance with Moses, the Innermost is the Ruach Elohim (the Spirit of God) who sowed the waters in the beginning of the world. He is the Sun King, our Divine Monad, the Alter-Ego of Cicerone." —Samael Aun Weor, *The Revolution of Beelzebub*

Kundalini: "Kundalini, the serpent power or mystic fire, is the primordial energy or Sakti that lies dormant or sleeping in the Muladhara Chakra, the centre of the body. It is called the serpentine or annular power on account of serpentine form. It is an electric fiery occult power, the great pristine force which underlies all organic and inorganic matter. Kundalini is the cosmic power in individual bodies. It is not a material force like electricity, magnetism, centripetal or centrifugal force. It is a spiritual potential Sakti or cosmic power. In reality it has no form. [...] O Divine Mother Kundalini, the Divine Cosmic Energy that is hidden in men! Thou art Kali, Durga, Adisakti, Rajarajeswari, Tripurasundari, Maha-Lakshmi, Maha-Sarasvati! Thou hast put on all these names and forms. Thou hast manifested as Prana, electricity, force, magnetism, cohesion, gravitation in this universe. This whole universe rests in Thy bosom. Crores of salutations unto thee. O Mother of this world! Lead me on to open the Sushumna Nadi and take Thee along the Chakras to Sahasrara Chakra and to merge myself in Thee and Thy consort, Lord

Siva. Kundalini Yoga is that Yoga which treats of Kundalini Sakti, the six centres of spiritual energy (Shat Chakras), the arousing of the sleeping Kundalini Sakti and its union with Lord Siva in Sahasrara Chakra, at the crown of the head. This is an exact science. This is also known as Laya Yoga. The six centres are pierced (Chakra Bheda) by the passing of Kundalini Sakti to the top of the head. 'Kundala' means 'coiled'. Her form is like a coiled serpent. Hence the name Kundalini." - Swami Sivananda, *Kundalini Yoga*

Logos: (Greek) means Verb or Word. In Greek and Hebrew metaphysics, the unifying principle of the world. The Logos is the manifested deity of every nation and people; the outward expression or the effect of the cause which is ever concealed. (Speech is the "logos" of thought). The Logos has three aspects, known universally as the Trinity or Trimurti. The First Logos is the Father, Brahma. The Second Logos is the Son, Vishnu. The Third Logos is the Holy Spirit, Shiva. One who incarnates the Logos becomes a Logos.

"The Logos is not an individual. The Logos is an army of ineffable beings." —Samael Aun Weor, *Sexology, the Basis of Endocrinology and Criminology*

Maithuna: Sanskrit, "sacramental intercourse."

The Sanskrit word Maithuna is used in Hindu Tantras (esoteric scriptures) to refer to the sacrament (sacred ritual) of sexual union between husband and wife.

Maithuna or Mithuna has various appearances
in scripture:

- Mithuna: paired, forming a pair; copulation;
  the zodiacal sign of Gemini in Vedic Astrology,
  which is depicted as a man and woman in a
  sexual embrace
- Mithunaya: to unite sexually
- Mithuni: to become paired, couple or united
  sexually

By means of the original Tantric Maithuna, after
being prepared psychologically and spiritually and initiated by a genuine teacher (guru),
the couple learns how to utilize their love and
spiritual aspiration in order to transform their
natural sexual forces to purify the mind, eliminate psychological defects, and awaken the latent
powers of the consciousness. The man represents
Shiva, the masculine aspect of the creative divine,
and the woman represents Shakti, the feminine
aspect and the source of the power of creation.

This method was kept in strictest secrecy for
thousands of years in order to preserve it in its
pure form, and to prevent crude-minded people
from deviating the teaching, other people, or
harming themselves. Nonetheless, some degenerated traditions (popularly called "left-hand" traditions, or black magic) interpret Maithuna or
sacramental sexuality according to their state of
degeneration, and use these sacred teachings to
justify their lust, desire, orgies, and other types
of deviations from pure, genuine Tantra.

Krishna: "And I am the strength of the strong,
devoid of lust and attachment. O best of the

Bharatas, I am sex not contrary to dharma."
(Bhagavad Gita 7.11)

Mantra: (Sanskrit, literally "mind protection") A
sacred word or sound. The use of sacred words
and sounds is universal throughout all religions
and mystical traditions, because the root of all
creation is in the Great Breath or the Word, the
Logos. "In the beginning was the Word..."

Meditation: "When the esotericist submerges himself into meditation, what he seeks is information." —Samael Aun Weor

"It is urgent to know how to meditate in order to
comprehend any psychic aggregate, or in other
words, any psychological defect. It is indispensable to know how to work with all our heart and
with all our soul, if we want the elimination to
occur." —Samael Aun Weor, *The Gnostic Bible: The
Pistis Sophia Unveiled*

"1. The Gnostic must first attain the ability to
stop the course of his thoughts, the capacity to
not think. Indeed, only the one who achieves
that capacity will hear the Voice of the Silence.

"2. When the Gnostic disciple attains the capacity to not think, then he must learn to concentrate his thoughts on only one thing.

"3. The third step is correct meditation. This
brings the first flashes of the new consciousness
into the mind.

"4. The fourth step is contemplation, ecstasy
or Samadhi. This is the state of Turiya (perfect
clairvoyance)." —Samael Aun Weor, *The Perfect
Matrimony*

Prana: (Sanskrit) Life-principle; the breath of life; energy. The vital breath, which sustains life in a physical body; the primal energy or force, of which other physical forces are manifestations. In the books of Yoga, prana is described as having five modifications, according to its five different functions. These are: prana (the vital energy that controls the breath), apana (the vital energy that carries downward unassimilated food and drink), samana (the vital energy that carries nutrition all over the body), vyama (the vital energy that pervades the entire body), and udana (the vital energy by which the contents of the stomach are ejected through the mouth). The word Prana is also used as a name of the Cosmic Soul, endowed with activity.

"Prana is the Great Breath. It is the Cosmic Christ. Prana is the life that palpitates within every atom, as it palpitates in every sun. Fire burns because of Prana. Water flows because of Prana. Wind blows because of Prana. The sun exists because of Prana; the life we have is Prana. Nothing can exist in the Universe without Prana. It is impossible for the most insignificant insect to be born, or for the smallest flower to bloom without Prana. Prana exists in the food that we eat, in the air that we breathe, and in the water that we drink. Prana exists within everything. When seminal energy is refined and totally transformed, the nervous system is provided with the richest type of Prana. This rich Prana is deposited within the brain in the form of pure Christic energy, the Wine of Light. An intimate connection exists between the mind, the Prana and the semen. We can gain domin-

ion over the mind and Prana by controlling the seminal energy with the force of willpower. Those people who spill the semen can never gain control over their mind, let alone Prana. Their efforts to gain control over their mind and over Prana will undoubtedly fail. People who gain sexual control, also gain control of their minds and control of their Prana. These types of human beings reach true liberation."
—Samael Aun Weor, *The Yellow Book*

"Prana is life and it circulates throughout all of our organs." "Prana circulates throughout all of our nadis and vital canals." "The sexual energy is Prana, life." "Prana is sexual. The sexual energy is solar. The solar energy is Christic. The Cosmic Christ is the Solar Logos. The solar energy comes from the Cosmic Christ. The Christic Prana makes the spike of wheat to grow; thus, the Christonic substance ready to be devoured remains enclosed within the grain. The water from the mountain glaciers penetrates within the stump to ripen the grape, within which the whole life, the whole Prana from the Sun-Christ remains enclosed." — Samael Aun Weor, *Kundalini Yoga*

Pranayama: (Sanskrit for "restraint [ayama] of energy, life force [prana]") A type of breathing exercise which transforms the life force (sexual energy) of the practitioner. There are many types of pranayama taught in the Gnostic tradition. You can learn some of them in the books *The Major Mysteries, Kundalini Yoga,* and *The Yellow Book.*

"Pranayama is a system of sexual transmutation for single persons." —Samael Aun Weor, *The Yellow Book*

Sadhana: (Sanskrit) "Instrument, means." A spiritual technique or method.

Sahaja Maithuna: (Sanskrit) Sanskrit: sahaja, "original, natural." Maithuna, "marriage, sacramental intercourse, a pair or one of each sex." A reference to superior sexuality in which the orgasm is abandoned and lust is replaced by love.

Samadhi: (Sanskrit) Literally means "union" or "combination" and its Tibetan equivalent means "adhering to that which is profound and definitive," or ting nge dzin, meaning "To hold unwaveringly, so there is no movement." Related terms include satori, ecstasy, manteia, etc. Samadhi is a state of consciousness. In the west, the term is used to describe an ecstatic state of consciousness in which the Essence escapes the painful limitations of the mind (the "I") and therefore experiences what is real: the Being, the Great Reality. There are many levels of Samadhi. In the sutras and tantras the term Samadhi has a much broader application whose precise interpretation depends upon which school and teaching is using it.

"Ecstasy is not a nebulous state, but a transcendental state of wonderment, which is associated with perfect mental clarity." —Samael Aun Weor, *The Elimination of Satan's Tail*

Sexual Magic: The word magic is derived from the ancient word magos "one of the members of the learned and priestly class," from O.Pers. magush, possibly from PIE *magh- "to be able, to have power." [Quoted from Online Etymology Dictionary].

"All of us possess some electrical and magnetic forces within, and, just like a magnet, we exert a force of attraction and repulsion... Between lovers that magnetic force is particularly powerful and its action has a far-reaching effect."
—Samael Aun Weor, *The Mystery of the Golden Blossom*

Sexual magic refers to an ancient science that has been known and protected by the purest, most spiritually advanced human beings, whose purpose and goal is the harnessing and perfection of our sexual forces. A more accurate translation of sexual magic would be "sexual priesthood." In ancient times, the priest was always accompanied by a priestess, for they represent the divine forces at the base of all creation: the masculine and feminine, the Yab-Yum, Ying-Yang, Father-Mother: the Elohim. Unfortunately, the term "sexual magic" has been grossly misinterpreted by mistaken persons such as Aleister Crowley, who advocated a host of degenerated practices, all of which belong solely to the lowest and most perverse mentality and lead only to the enslavement of the consciousness, the worship of lust and desire, and the decay of humanity. True, upright, heavenly sexual magic is the natural harnessing of our latent forces, making them active and harmonious with nature and the divine, and which leads to the perfection of the human being.

"People are filled with horror when they hear about sexual magic; however, they are not filled with horror when they give themselves to all kinds of sexual perversion and to all kinds of carnal passion." —Samael Aun Weor, *The Perfect Matrimony*

Shiva: (Sanskrit शिव) A multifaceted symbol in the Hindu pantheon.

"Lord Siva is the pure, changeless, attributeless, all-pervading transcendental consciousness.... At the end of Pralaya, the Supreme Lord thinks of re-creation of the world. He is then known by the name Sadasiva. He is the root-cause of creation. From Sadasiva creation begins... [Additionally,] Lord Siva represents the destructive aspect of Brahman... He destroys all bondage, limitation and sorrow of His devotees. He is the giver of Mukti or the final emancipation. He is the universal Self. He is the true Self of all creatures. He is the dweller in the cremation-ground, in the region of the dead, those who are dead to the world. The Jivas and the world originate from Him, exist in Him, are sustained and rejected by Him and are ultimately merged in Him. He is the support, source and substratum of the whole world. He is an embodiment of Truth, Beauty, Goodness and Bliss. He is Satyam, Sivam, Subham, Sundaram, Kantam. He is the God of gods, Deva-Deva. He is the Great Deity—Mahadeva." —Swami Sivananda, *Lord Siva and His Worship*

The Hindu creator and destroyer, the third aspect of the Trimurti (Brahma, Vishnu, Shiva). The Third Logos. The Holy Spirit. The sexual force. The sephirah Binah. Symbolized by a linga / lingum, a male sexual organ.

Solar Bodies: The physical, vital, astral, mental, and causal bodies that are created through the beginning stages of Alchemy/Tantra and that provide a basis for existence in their corresponding levels of nature, just as the physical body does in the physical world. These bodies or vehicles are superior due to being created out of Solar (Christic) Energy, as opposed to the inferior, lunar bodies we receive from nature. Also known as the Wedding Garment (Christianity), the Merkabah (Kabbalah), To Soma Heliakon (Greek), and Sahu (Egyptian).

"All the Masters of the White Lodge, the Angels, Archangels, Thrones, Seraphim, Virtues, etc., etc., etc. are garbed with the Solar Bodies. Only those who have Solar Bodies have the Being incarnated. Only someone who possesses the Being is an authentic Human Being." —Samael Aun Weor, *The Esoteric Treatise of Hermetic Astrology*

Third Logos: The creative aspect of the divine trinity of forces that originates all things (see: Logos). In Hebrew, this aspect is called בינה Binah, which means "understanding." Binah is the third sephirah on the Kabbalistic Tree of Life. In other religions, this aspect of divinity is known as:

Aztec: Tlaloc Quetzalcoatl

Christian: The Holy Spirit

Egyptian: Osiris-Isis

Gnostic: The Third Logos; The 8th Aeon

Hindu: Shiva

Mayan: Raxa Kakulha

Nordic: Thor

The Third Logos is related to:

Body: Nirmanakaya

Dimension: Seventh or Zero Dimension

Heaven of: Saturn and Jupiter

Level of Consciousness: Nirmanakaya (Buddhist), Aralim (Kabbalah), Thrones

Vital Body: (Also called Ethereal Body) The superior aspect of the physical body, composed of the energy or vital force that provides life to the physical body.

"It is written that the vital body or the foundation of organic life within each one of us has four ethers. The chemical ether and the ether of life are related with chemical processes and sexual reproduction. The chemical ether is a specific foundation for the organic chemical phenomena. The ether of life is the foundation of the reproductive and transformative sexual processes of the race. The two superior ethers, luminous and reflective, have more elevated functions. The luminous ether is related with the caloric, luminous, perceptive, etc., phenomena. The reflective ether serves as a medium of expression for willpower and imagination." —Samael Aun Weor, *The Gnostic Bible: The Pistis Sophia Unveiled*

In Tibetan Buddhism, the vital body is known as the subtle body (lus phra-mo). In Hinduism, it is known as pranamayakosa.

White Fraternity, Lodge, or Brotherhood: That ancient collection of pure souls who maintain the highest and most sacred of sciences: White Magic or White Tantra. It is called White due to its purity and cleanliness. This "Brotherhood" or "Lodge" includes human beings of the highest order from every race, culture, creed and religion, and of both sexes.

Yoga: (Sanskrit) "union." Similar to the Latin "religare," the root of the word "religion." In Tibetan, it is "rnal-'byor" which means "union with the fundamental nature of reality."

"The word YOGA comes from the root Yuj which means to join, and in its spiritual sense, it is that process by which the human spirit is brought into near and conscious communion with, or is merged in, the Divine Spirit, according as the nature of the human spirit is held to be separate from (Dvaita, Visishtadvaita) or one with (Advaita) the Divine Spirit." —Swami Sivananda, *Kundalini Yoga*

"Patanjali defines Yoga as the suspension of all the functions of the mind. As such, any book on Yoga, which does not deal with these three aspects of the subject, viz., mind, its functions and the method of suspending them, can he safely laid aside as unreliable and incomplete." —Swami Sivananda, *Practical Lessons In Yoga*

"The word yoga means in general to join one's mind with an actual fact..." —The 14th Dalai Lama

"The soul aspires for the union with his Innermost, and the Innermost aspires for the union with his Glorian." —Samael Aun Weor, *The Revolution of Beelzebub*

"All of the seven schools of Yoga are within Gnosis, yet they are in a synthesized and absolutely practical way. There is Tantric Hatha Yoga in the practices of the Maithuna (Sexual Magic). There is practical Raja Yoga in the work with the chakras. There is Gnana Yoga in our practices and mental disciplines which we have cultivated in secrecy for millions of years. We have Bhakti Yoga in our prayers and Rituals. We have Laya Yoga in our meditation and respiratory exercises. Samadhi exists in our practices with the Maithuna and during our deep meditations. We live the path of Karma Yoga in our upright actions, in our upright thoughts, in our upright feelings, etc." —Samael Aun Weor, *The Revolution of Beelzebub*

"The Yoga that we require today is actually ancient Gnostic Christian Yoga, which absolutely rejects the idea of Hatha Yoga. We do not recommend Hatha Yoga simply because, spiritually speaking, the acrobatics of this discipline are fruitless; they should be left to the acrobats of the circus." —Samael Aun Weor, *The Yellow Book*

"Yoga has been taught very badly in the Western world. Multitudes of pseudo-sapient yogis have spread the false belief that the true yogi must be an infrasexual (an enemy of sex). Some of these false yogis have never even visited India; they are infrasexual pseudo-yogis. These ignoramuses believe that they are going to achieve in-depth realization only with the yogic exercises, such as asanas, pranayamas, etc. Not only do they have such false beliefs, but what is worse is that they propagate them; thus, they misguide many people away from the difficult, straight, and narrow door that leads unto the light. No authentically initiated yogi from India would ever think that he could achieve his inner Self-realization with pranayamas or asanas, etc. Any legitimate yogi from India knows very well that such yogic exercises are only co-assistants that are very useful for their health and for the development of their powers, etc. Only the Westerners and pseudo-yogis have within their minds the belief that they can achieve Self-realization with such exercises. Sexual Magic is practiced very secretly within the ashrams of India. Any true yogi initiate from India works with the Arcanum A.Z.F. This is taught by the great yogis from India that have visited the Western world, and if it has not been taught by these great, initiated Hindustani yogis, if it has not been published in their books of yoga, it was in order to avoid scandals. You can be absolutely sure that the yogis who do not practice Sexual Magic will never achieve birth in the superior worlds. Thus, whosoever affirms the contrary is a liar, an impostor." —Samael Aun Weor, *Alchemy and Kabbalah in the Tarot*

About the Author

His name is Hebrew סמאל און ואור, and is pronounced "sam-ayel on vay-or." You may not have heard of him, but Samael Aun Weor changed the world.

In 1950, in his first two books, he became the first person to reveal the esoteric secret hidden in all the world's great religions, and for that, accused of "healing the ill," he was put in prison. Nevertheless, he did not stop. Between 1950 and 1977 – merely twenty-seven years – not only did Samael Aun Weor write over sixty books on the most difficult subjects in the world, such as consciousness, kabbalah, physics, tantra, meditation, etc., in which he deftly exposed the singular root of all knowledge — which he called Gnosis — he simultaneously inspired millions of people across the entire span of Latin America: stretching across twenty countries and an area of more than 21,000,000 kilometers, founding schools everywhere, even in places without electricity or post offices.

During those twenty-seven years, he experienced all the extremes that humanity could give him, from adoration to death threats, and in spite of the enormous popularity of his books and lectures, he renounced an income, refused recognitions, walked away from accolades, and consistently turned away those who would worship him. He held as friends both presidents and peasants, and yet remained a mystery to all.

When one reflects on the effort and will it requires to perform even day to day tasks, it is astonishing to consider the herculean efforts required to accomplish what he did in such a short time. But, there is a reason: he was a man who knew who he was, and what he had to do. A true example of compassion and selfless service, Samael Aun Weor dedicated the whole of his life to freely helping anyone and everyone find the path out of suffering. His mission was to show all of humanity the universal source of all spiritual traditions, which he did not only through his writings and lectures, but also through his actions.

Your book reviews matter.

Glorian Publishing is a very small non-profit organization, thus we have no money to spend on marketing and advertising. Fortunately, there is a proven way to gain the attention of readers: book reviews. Mainstream book reviewers won't review these books, but you can.

The path of liberation requires the daily balance of three active factors:

- · birth of virtue
- · death of vice
- · sacrifice for others

Writing book reviews is a powerful way to sacrifice for others. By writing book reviews on popular websites, you help to make the books more visible to humanity, and you might help save a soul from suffering. Will you do your part to help us show these wonderful teachings to others? Take a moment today to write a review.

Donate

Glorian Publishing is a 501(c)3 non-profit organization dedicated to spreading the sacred universal doctrine to suffering humanity. All of our works are made possible by the kindness and generosity of sponsors. If you would like to make a tax-deductible donation, you may send it to the address below, or visit our website for other alternatives. If you would like to sponsor the publication of a book, please contact us at (844) 945-6742 or help@gnosticteachings.org.

Glorian Publishing
PO Box 110225
Brooklyn, NY 11211 US
Phone: (844) 945-6742
VISIT US ONLINE AT gnosticteachings.org